Bone Metastasis and Molecular Mechanisms

Cancer Metastasis – Biology and Treatment

VOLUME 6

Titles published in this Series are:

Volume 1: Cancer Metastasis, Molecular and Cellular Mechanisms and Clinical Intervention.
Editors: Wen G. Jiang and Robert E. Mansel.
ISBN 0-7923-6395-7

Volume 2: Growth Factors and Receptors in Cancer Metastasis.
Editors: Wen G. Jiang, Kunio Matsumoto and Toshikazu Nakamura.
ISBN 0-7923-7141-0

Volume 3: Cancer Metastasis-Related Genes
Editor: Danny R. Welch
ISBN 1-4020-0522-9

Volume 4: Proteases and Their Inhibitors in Cancer Metastasis
Editor: Jean-Michel Foidart and Ruth J. Muschel
ISBN 1-4020-0923-2

Volume 5: Micrometastasis
Editor: Klaus Pantel
ISBN 1-4020-1155-5

Bone Metastasis and Molecular Mechanisms

Pathophysiology

Edited by

Gurmit Singh
Director of Research, Juravinski Cancer Centre/
Professor of Pathology & Molecular Medicine,
McMaster University, Hamilton, Ontario, Canada

and

William Orr
Chair, Department of Pathology, University of Manitoba,
Winnipeg, Manitoba, Canada

KLUWER ACADEMIC PUBLISHERS
DORDRECHT / BOSTON / LONDON

A C.I.P. Catalogue record for this book is available from the Library of Congress.

ISBN 1-4020-1984-X

Published by Kluwer Academic Publishers,
P.O. Box 17, 3300 AA Dordrecht, The Netherlands.

Sold and distributed in North, Central and South America
by Kluwer Academic Publishers,
101 Philip Drive, Norwell, MA 02061, U.S.A.

In all other countries, sold and distributed
by Kluwer Academic Publishers,
P.O. Box 322, 3300 AH Dordrecht, The Netherlands.

Printed on acid-free paper

Printed in the Netherlands.

Dedicated to:

Bone Metastasis Researchers and Cancer Patients.

CONTENTS

CONTRIBUTORS

EDITORS

Gurmit Singh
Director of Research
Juravinski Cancer Centre
Professor of Pathology and Molecular Medicine
McMaster University
Hamilton, Ontario, Canada

William F. Orr
Chair of Pathology
Health Sciences Center
University of Manitoba
Winnipeg, Manitoba, Canada

CONTRIBUTORS

Robin L. Anderson
Head, Cancer Biology Laboratory
Peter MacCallum Cancer Institute
East Melbourne, Victoria, Australia

Nicholas A. Athanasou
Departments of Surgery and Pathology
Nuffield Department of Orthopaedic Surgery
University of Oxford
Oxford, UK

Andrew Belch
University of Alberta and Cross Cancer Institute
Alberta, Canada

Paolo Bianco
Dipartmeento di Medicina Sperimentale e Patologia
Universita "La Sapeinza"
Parco Scientifico Biomedico San Raffaele
Rome, Italy

Jeroen Buijs
Department of Endocrinology
Leiden University Medical Center
Leiden, Netherlands

Wilhelmina C.M Duivenvoorden
Northwestern Ontario Regional Cancer Centre
Thunder Bay, Ontario, Canada

Bedrick L. Eckhardt
Peter MacCallum Cancer Centre
East Melbourne, Victoria, Australia

Thomas H. Hassard
Department of Community Health Science
University of Manitoba
Winnipeg, Manitoba, Canada

Paul J. Kostenuik
Research Scientist
Amgen Inc.
Thousand Oaks, California, USA

Mary Mackenzie
Medical Oncology
Juravinski Cancer Centre
Hamilton, Ontario, Canada

Pierre P. Major
Medical Oncology
Juravinski Cancer Centre
Hamilton, Ontario, Canada

Andrew P. Mazar
Attenuon, LLC
San Diego, California, USA

Belinda S. Parker
Peter MacCallum Cancer Center
East Melbourne, Victoria, Australia

Linda M. Pilarski
University of Alberta and Cross Cancer Institute
Alberta, Canada

Patrick M. Pilarski
University of Alberta and Cross Cancer Institute
Alberta, Canada

Shafaat A. Rabbani
Departments of Physiology and Medicine
Royal Victoria Hospital
McGill University Health Centre
Montreal, Quebec, Canada

Martin Reed
Department of Radiology
Health Sciences Center
Winnipeg, Manitoba, Canada

Tony Reiman
University of Alberta and Cross Cancer Institute
Alberta, Canada

Mara Riminucci
Parco Scientifico Biomedico San Raffaele
Rome Italy
Departmento di Medicina Sperimentale
Universita dell'Aquila
L'Aquila, Italy

Pamela Gehron Robey
Craniofacial and Skeletal Diseases Branch
National Institute of Dental and Craniofacial Research
National Institutes of Health
Department of Health and Human Services
Bethesda, Maryland, USA

Eric Seidlitz
Department of Research
Juravinski Cancer Centre
Hamilton, Ontario, Canada

Julie A. Sharp
Department of Surgery
University of Melbourne
St. Vincent's Institute of Medical Research
Fitzroy, Australia

Jonathan C. Sharp
Institute for Biodiagnostics
National Research Council of Canada
Winnipeg, Manitoba, Canada

Nicholas Shukeir
Departments of Physiology and Medicine
Royal Victoria Hospital
McGill University Health Centre
Montreal, Quebec, Canada

Sadmeet Singh
Department of Research
Juravinski Cancer Centre
Hamilton, Ontario, Canada

James A. Thliveris
Department of Human Anatomy and Cell Science
University of Manitoba
Winnipeg, Manitoba, Canada

Erik W. Thompson
University of Melbourne
Department of Surgery
St. Vincent's Institute of Medical Research
Bernard O'Brien Institute of Microsurgery
St. Vincent's Hospital
Fitzroy, Australia

Gabri Van Der Pluijm
Leiden University Medical Center
Department of Endocrinology
Leiden, Netherlands

Snezana Vikmirovic-Popovic
Department of Research
Juravinski Cancer Centre
Hamilton, Ontario, Canada

Michael H. Weber
Department of Pathology
University of Manitoba
Institute for Biodiagnostics
National Research Council of Canada
Winnipeg, Manitoba, Canada

PREFACE

Bone is a frequent site for metastasis in patients with carcinomas of the breast, lung and prostate and hematopoietic malignancies. They result in significant clinical morbidity and are usually related to extensive tumor-associated osteolysis. Despite the magnitude of this problem, the current therapies have had variable success. The tumor cells relationship with host tissue is a major factor in their ability to develop into macroscopic metastases. The "seed" and "soil" hypothesis of metastasis was proposed in Paget's paper of 1889 discussing the distribution of metastasis in breast cancer. Unraveling the molecular mechanisms governing the interaction between the host microenvironment and tumour cell is key to the development of new therapies to deal with metastases.

This multi-authored book focuses specially on the pathophysiology of bone metastases. The writers are all active investigators with research programs on bone metastasis and leaders in the field. They have reviewed the current literature in their areas of research. The first chapter by Dr. Robin Anderson's group discusses various models of breast cancer metastasis. Chapter 2 from Dr. Erik Thompson's group is focused on the quantitation aspects of bone metastasis. Chapters 3 and 4 from Dr. Gurmit Singh and Dr. Bill Orr's group have outlined comparative morphometric techniques to study bone metastasis and clinical modalities for the diagnosis of bone metastasis. Chapter 5, 6, 7 and 8 have a theme on the microenvironment and associated pathophysiologies of bone metastasis. In chapter 5, Dr. Pamela Robey has outlined the metastasis in the bone marrow environment. Dr. Athanasou evaluates the role of tumor-associated macrophages in chapter 6. The relationship between malignant cells and the bone macroenvironment is discussed in chapter 7 by Dr. Linda Pilarski's group. Networking via angiogenesis and lymphangiogenesis is highlighted in chapter 8 by Dr. Gabri Van Der Pluijm's group.

Chapters 9, 10, 11, 12 and 13 relate to key areas in the development of new therapies for bone metastasis. In chapter 9, Dr. Shafaat Rabbani's group has outlined an approach to developing novel therapeutic intervention using prostate cancer models. In chapter 10, Dr. Gurmit Singh's group provides a unique opportunity of using osteotropic agents in the treatment of bone metastasis. Dr. Paul Kostenuik discusses the role of OPG in pathobiology of osteolysis and potential use as a therapeutic agent. Chapter 12 discusses the role of matrix metalloproteinases in bone metastasis and potential therapeutic targets. Finally in chapter 13 Drs. Pierre Major and Mary Mackenzie provide a rational for the use of bisphosphonates in bone metastasis.

This is a comprehensive treatise to the subject of bone metastasis as it pertains to the pathophysiology and mechanisms of bone metastasis. The authors and editors hope this book will help in furthering fundamental research in bone metastasis.

The editors would like to thank all the contributing authors and congratulate them for their scholarly efforts in the preparation of these chapters, which have summarized current literature in their field. We would also like to thank Dr. Richard Ablin and Wen Jiang for inviting us to edit a volume on bone metastasis for the book series on Cancer Metastasis: Biology and Treatment. We would like to acknowledge assistance from the Publishing Editor, Dr. Cristina Miranda Alves dos Santos and her assistant Ms. Melania Ruiz Esparza from Kluwer press. Finally the support and assistance of Mrs. Pauline Hiltz and Ms. Heather Blackborow is greatly appreciated.

Professor Gurmit Singh

Chapter 1

MODELS OF BREAST CANCER METASTASIS TO BONE: CHARACTERIZATION OF A CLINICALLY RELEVANT MODEL

Belinda S. Parker, Bedrich L. Eckhardt and Robin L. Anderson
Peter MacCallum Cancer Centre, St. Andrews Place, East Melbourne, Victoria, Australia

1. BREAST CANCER: THE CLINICAL PROBLEM

Breast cancer metastasis to the skeleton is a severe clinical problem that occurs in 70% of patients with advanced disease. Bone is also a frequent site of metastasis of some other cancers, including prostate. Bone metastases in breast cancer are predominantly osteolytic due to the resorption of bone following excessive activation of osteoclasts. This leads to major clinical problems including severe pain, hypercalcemia, bone fractures and nerve-compression syndromes (1).

When diagnosed early, breast cancer can be treated successfully, but the advanced disease is difficult to control and chances of survival are much reduced. Treatment of patients with bone involvement is essentially palliative, aiming primarily to minimize pain and other debilitating clinical symptoms, rather than to affect a cure. Due to the severe morbidity of this disease, there is an urgent need for new treatment options. Bone metastases are difficult to treat for several reasons. First, invasion and release of tumor cells into the circulation has often occurred before detection and removal of the primary tumor. Second, the heterogeneity of the primary cancer leads to difficulties in identifying factors that are predictive of metastasis and therefore potential targets for therapy (2). Finally, there is a lack of an understanding of the molecular interactions that take place in the bone

G. Singh and W. Orr (eds.), Bone Metastasis and Molecular Mechanisms, 1-18.

microenvironment. The search for the best therapeutic targets to block metastasis to bone is hampered by the lack of clinically relevant *in vivo* models of breast cancer metastasis. Identification of genes that are clinically relevant in metastasis to bone is required to shift therapy from palliative to specific and effective treatments. The next section will cover what is known about the steps involved in the metastatic cascade and which of these steps are potential targets for preventing the growth of metastases in bone.

2. MECHANISMS AND POTENTIAL THERAPEUTIC TARGETS FOR METASTASIS TO BONE

The metastatic cascade begins with growth and invasion of the primary tumor and progresses to the formation of macrometastases at distant sites. It is evident that this process involves interactions between the tumor cells, the surrounding stroma and the blood vessels that provide factors essential both for tumor growth and for dissemination of tumor cells (3). Interactions with the stroma are required for the survival and growth of breast cancer cells at specific secondary sites, such as bone. A number of theories have been proposed to explain the increased colonization of tumor cells at specific secondary sites. These theories, including Paget's "seed and soil" hypothesis, the "circulation" theory and the "homing" theory, have been extensively reviewed in the past (4, 5) and will not be discussed here. Several studies have demonstrated a contribution by all three theories, in that the release of cells into the circulation and their arrest may be random or in some cases controlled by a chemotactic homing mechanism (6) but the attachment, survival and growth into macrometastases at secondary sites is specific to stromal interactions within that organ.

Steps involved in metastasis include growth of the primary tumor, loss of cell-cell adhesion, invasion into surrounding stroma, intravasation into the circulation and arrest at a secondary site, either randomly or by specific interaction with vascular endothelial cells. Tumor cells then extravasate from vessels, form micrometastases and later macrometastases if there is a suitable microenvironment (7, 8).

Recent *in vivo* imaging studies have suggested that cells within the circulation extravasate efficiently and somewhat randomly at secondary sites. The rate-limiting step was proposed to be the formation of macrometastatic lesions, with the majority of cells never achieving this step (9). Most cells that extravasate into a secondary tissue die or remain dormant (10). However, a few tumor cells initiate favorable interactions with the stroma, promoting their survival and growth. It is of great interest to understand the specific molecular characteristics that allow these few cells to initiate the process of tumor growth and bone resorption, a process termed the "vicious cycle" (11). Factors released by tumor cells stimulate osteoclast activation either directly or through osteoblasts leading to bone lysis and release of tumor growth stimulating factors from the bone matrix.

What is the difference between the gene expression profiles of cells that remain dormant and those that can progress to form macrometastatic lesions? It has been postulated that the latter may have the ability to escape immune recognition by expressing a subset of surface proteins that are also expressed by normal cells in the bone environment (12). Could this explain why many of the cells do not die, but remain dormant? Alternatively, could the niche within the bone marrow where a tumor cell lodges after extravasation dictate its future growth capacity? The ability of the tumor cells to interact with bone stromal cells to stimulate angiogenesis is likely to be another important regulator of bone metastasis.

To date, there are few therapies available to block the growth of bone metastases (11, 13). Since the rate-limiting step is likely to be growth at the secondary site, it may be more logical to target this step rather than the initial release of tumor cells into the circulation. The most attractive therapies are those that prevent tumor cell attachment and communication with stromal cells in bone, or that prevent activation of bone-derived growth factors required for bone resorption or that inhibit angiogenesis. Thus, new therapies need to be directed at specific targets in the cell. The rational way to identify these therapeutic agents is to determine the molecular mechanisms that provide tumor cells with the ability to initiate bone destruction. This approach requires the utilization and further development of good models of bone metastasis. One class of compounds that have been shown to interfere with bone resorption is the bisphosphonates. As well as blocking bone resorption, the bisphosphonates inhibit tumor cell attachment to bone, inhibit activity of MMPs and promote apoptosis of tumor cells (14, 15). It is important to determine the specific mechanism of action of the bisphosphonates to aid in the search for analogs with enhanced activity. Clinically relevant models of metastasis to bone are needed for complete analysis of therapeutic potential. These models can also be used to measure the efficacy of these new therapies in combination with other anti-cancer agents, especially since patient survival is not always improved by bisphosphonate treatment alone (14, 16, 17). However, treatment with bisphosphonates before the onset of bone metastases has been shown to reduce metastatic onset and prolong patient survival (18).

Another promising therapy that needs to be tested in more clinically relevant models of malignant bone disease is osteoprotegerin (OPG), a soluble decoy receptor for RANK ligand, which is a TNF-related protein released by osteoblasts to trigger activation of osteoclasts. Preclinical studies indicate that OPG is effective in inhibition of osteolysis caused by tumor cells (19, 20).

The interactions between tumor cells and bone stroma that initiate the cycle of bone destruction and tumor growth are critical for understanding the bone metastatic process (21). Although there have been studies of tumor cell growth in the bone environment (22, 23), the biology/pathogenesis of bone metastasis is still not well understood due to the lack of models that mimic the entire process of breast cancer metastasis.

It is likely that expression of a number of genes in the primary tumor and/or in the bone microenvironment will be important for the development of osteolytic bone metastases (7, 8, 11, 23). Those already identified as potentially important include parathyroid hormone-related protein (PTHrP) (a major contributor to bone resorption that will be discussed in more detail later in the chapter), interleukin-11 (IL-11) and IL-6, which have been shown to stimulate bone resorption and may (like PTHrP) induce osteolysis (24), calcitonin receptors, the bone proteins osteopontin and bone sialoprotein (25), tumor necrosis factor-α (TNFα) (26), transforming growth factor-β (TGF-β) (27), prostaglandins (28), receptor activator of NF-κB ligand, (RANKL) (29), macrophage-colony stimulating factor (M-CSF) (29, 30) and human platelet derived growth factor-BB (hPDGF-BB) (31). A number of other genes have been shown to be involved in the metastatic process, but are not specific to bone metastasis such as E-cadherin, VEGF, uPA (32), αvβ3 integrin (33), maspin (34), matrix metalloproteinases (MMPs) (35) and other proteases that may aid in invasion. There are now over twenty MMPs identified and it is likely that specific MMPs will be required for local invasion and release of cells from the primary tumor whilst others are active at different sites of metastasis. This remains an important aspect of metastasis that has not been thoroughly investigated.

Although many of the above mentioned candidate genes are differentially expressed in secondary bone tumors compared to primary tumors, a single accurate predictor to identify patients who will develop bone disease is still lacking.

3. MODELS OF METASTASIS TO BONE

An obstacle for research on bone metastasis is the lack of patient samples, since bone metastatic lesions are rarely removed surgically. In cases where the lesion is removed, access to a sample of the matching primary tumor is unlikely to be available due to the time delay between primary tumor onset and metastatic occurrence. It is therefore very difficult to compare primary and metastatic lesions from the same patient. Archival samples are useful for genetic screens and *in situ* hybridisation or immunohistochemical techniques for expression analysis of selected genes. However, if a gene is found to have altered expression, it is very difficult to determine its function, whether it promotes or suppresses metastasis or whether it is downstream from the effector gene. It is also difficult to analyze the effectiveness of specific treatments to target the activity of the gene. Obviously the preferred approach is a model that can be utilized for genetic screens and is amenable for functional studies. Good models are not only important for a study of breast cancer pathogenesis and gene function but also for assessing the activity and potential of new therapies prior to patient administration.

Many current animal models of metastasis are not ideal for functional studies or drug testing since they do not encompass the whole metastatic process from primary tumor formation to growth of bone metastatic lesions. Very few metastasis models spontaneously metastasize to bone, most only mimic the latter stages of bone metastasis. It must therefore be questioned whether the results obtained from these experimental metastasis models are relevant to the complete process in breast cancer patients. However, despite their limitations, the commonly used experimental models have yielded much of our current knowledge of metastasis to bone, as summarized below.

3.1 Xenograft Metastasis Models

Xenograft models have been used extensively for studying bone metastasis *in vivo*, and have been useful in determining the genes from both tumor epithelium and bone stroma that regulate bone resorption. These models involve injection of human tumor cells into immunocompromised mice. Common avenues for injection are subcutaneous sites, the mammary gland, directly into bone, the left ventricle of the heart and the tail vein.

Subcutaneous or orthotopic injections of human breast cancer cells into the mammary fat pad of immunocompromised mice have not been of value in the study of bone metastasis. Injection of tumor cells into these sites leads to growth of primary tumors that rarely metastasize except to draining lymph nodes and occasionally to lung. However, it has been reported recently that MDA-MB-435 human breast tumor cells can be isolated from lung and bone of SCID mice bearing a mammary fat pad tumor that is excised 8 weeks after tumor cell inoculation (36).

The injection of cells directly into bone (37) lacks both formation of a primary tumor and the process of entry and exit from the circulation, and it is also likely that such an injection will cause injury at the site of injection, leading to a local inflammatory response. However, this route of injection is useful for the investigation of tumor growth in the bone environment.

Tail vein injections result in lung metastases (38) but rarely lead to the formation of bone metastases. As with the mammary fat pad injections, this may be due to the rapid progression of tumor growth in the lungs of these mice leading to death prior to skeletal involvement, or due to the lung being the first capillary bed for arrest of cells. However, bone seeking MDA-MB-231 clones that have been selected *in vivo* for preferential dissemination to bone, expand and form osteolytic lesions after tail vein injection (39).

The most common model that has been utilized for analysis of bone metastases in breast cancer is injection of MDA-MB-231 human breast cancer cells into the left ventricle of the heart of immunocompromised mice (40). The cells metastasize predominantly to bone and occasionally to brain, ovary and adrenal glands (41). The MDA-MB-231 intracardiac model triggers osteolytic damage in bone, which correlates with the extent of tumor burden (42). This model has enabled numerous studies of the role of specific genes in breast cancer growth in the bone environment. By multiple cycles of injection and recovery of cells from bone, Yoneda and colleagues (43) selected bone seeking clones that retained a similar tumorigenicity to the parental cell line yet metastasized specifically to bone. These clones formed larger osteolytic lesions and expressed increased amounts of PTHrP compared to the parental line.

Although the intracardiac model has provided valuable information on the interactions of tumor cells with bone stroma and the factors involved in osteolysis, there are disadvantages in using this model to study metastatic breast cancer. Three of these disadvantages are:

1. the lack of a primary tumor
2. the introduction of a bolus of circulating cells
3. the use of mice lacking a competent immune system.

In a model lacking a primary tumor, it is difficult to ascertain if the gene expression changes that are found in experimental bone metastases will be relevant when looking at the metastatic process as a whole. It is not possible to show that a gene that seems to be important for secondary tumor growth and/or bone resorption is also expressed in the primary tumor and if it is, whether its expression correlates with the incidence of distant metastasis and hence patient survival. Also, analysis of the processes of migration and invasion in tissue culture or in model systems where no primary tumors are formed, ignores the contribution of tumor-associated stromal cells to motility and invasion of tumor cells from the primary site.

In the pathogenesis of breast cancer metastasis, cells are released from the primary site and enter the circulation in small numbers over a long period of time. It is not known what differences a large bolus of cells will cause, but it can be hypothesized that cell migration and arrest in distant capillary beds may be influenced. It must also be recognized that the tissue culture cells used for intracardiac injection have not been adapted to *in vivo* growth and selection prior to release into the vasculature.

The immune system can modulate tumor growth and metastasis in both a positive and negative way. Inflammatory cells and various cytokines have been shown to promote metastasis. For example, tumor associated macrophages (TAMs) have a role in progression at both primary and secondary tumor sites. Recent studies have indicated that TAMs promote breast tumor growth (44). There is also a role for cytokines in osteoclastic bone resorption as indicated recently by the finding that chemokines, macrophage inflammatory protein 1-α (MIP-1α) and -β (MIP-1β), are present in bone marrow of patients with active myeloma bone disease and increase osteoclast formation (45, 46). Belonging to the RANTES family, these chemokines act as chemoattractants and activators of monocytes, from which osteoclasts are derived.

Other cells of the immune system, such as cytotoxic T lymphocytes (CTL) and natural killer (NK) cells recognize and kill tumor cells (47, 48). CTL are substantially depleted in nude and SCID mice, thus allowing growth of allogeneic tumor cells. In syngeneic hosts, tumor cells have been reported to undergo changes that allow their escape from immune surveillance. Loss or alteration of the MHC class 1 phenotype will provide a survival advantage to cells, allowing them to escape recognition and killing by CTL and NK cells and consequently develop as metastases (49, 50). A recent study investigated the MHC class 1 phenotype in disseminated tumor cells in bone marrow of patient samples and found a positive association between down regulation of MHC class 1 and unfavorable outcome (49). Thus the loss of MHC class 1 expression may play a role in allowing tumor cells to form bone metastatic lesions, such phenotypic differences thereby defining the cells that can form metastatic lesions. In the absence of a competent immune system, discrimination between cells based on MHC class 1 expression does not occur. Additionally, it has been reported that cells may express specific proteins on their surface to escape host immune surveillance (12, 51-53).

Whilst metastasis models utilizing immunodeficient mice do not consider these important aspects of metastasis, they remain the only way of studying human tumor growth and metastasis in mice.

3.2 Transgenic Mice

Transgenic models of breast cancer express oncogenes specifically targeted to the mammary gland by use of mammary specific promoters such as whey acidic protein (WAP), rat prostatic steroid binding protein (C(3)1) (54) and mouse mammary tumor virus (MMTV) (55). Transgenic models have considerable advantages over transplantable models in that tumor initiation closely resembles the early events in human cancer. Transgenic mice enable questions to be asked about the contribution of specific genes to tumorigenesis in mammary epithelium. The WAP-TAg (WAP-Simian Virus (SV) 40 T antigen) oncogenic mice are a useful background model of tumor initiation, developing mammary tumors with 100% frequency, and can be used for crossing to transgenic mice bearing a gene of interest to determine its role in tumor progression. An example of such a cross is with WAP-maspin transgenic mice that revealed the role of maspin in inhibiting tumor growth *in* vivo (56). The MMTV promoter system has been used to demonstrate that expression of a number of genes, including the human oncogenes myc (57) and Wnt-1 (58), can cause mammary cancer in mice, as in humans. A similar result was found with the mammary-specific knockout of the tumor suppressor gene BRCA1 (59). However, whilst transgenic models are valuable for studies of both mammary development and the molecular pathways of mammary cancer initiation and progression, no models exist that encompass metastasis to bone. When genes important for metastasis to bone have been identified, it will be possible to return to these transgenic models and cross the mice to strains bearing mammary gland specific expression of one of these genes, thus generating a transgenic model of breast cancer metastasis to bone.

4. PARATHYROID HORMONE RELATED PROTEIN (PTHRP) AND BONE METASTASIS

Studies, largely using the MDA-MB-231 intracardiac model, have found a number of genes that are altered in breast tumors and that appear to have a role in breast cancer progression. One gene that has received considerable attention due to its role in bone biology is PTHrP (60). PTHrP was originally identified as a causal agent of humoral hypercalcemia of malignancy (HHM) (61, 62). It stimulates osteoclastic bone resorption and is present in all patients with HHM and in 75% of patients with breast carcinoma metastatic to bone, but is not detected in normal plasma (63). Studies utilizing the MDA-MB-231 intracardiac model indicate that PTHrP over-expression leads to enhanced bone disease and conversely, that reduced PTHrP expression inhibits bone metastases (60, 64). These data indicate that PTHrP may have an important role in metastatic disease (aside from hypercalcemia), as a mediator of bone destruction and has led to the proposal that it could be utilized as a predictive marker in primary tumors of subsequent bone metastasis. This has been confirmed in some studies (65-67) but has not been confirmed in a large prospective study published recently (68). Here, it was shown that PTHrP is associated with a less invasive phenotype and that PTHrP expression in the primary tumor correlates with a reduced incidence of bone metastasis. The discrepancy between experimental studies using the MDA-MB-231 intracardiac model and the clinical data remains unexplained but reveals the importance of using clinically relevant models to study metastasis. Such a model is now available (see below), and has revealed that PTHrP expression in the primary tumor was not a predictor of bone metastasis (Tavaria et al., submitted for publication). Further, it was shown recently that whilst chemically induced mammary tumors in mice over-expressing PTHrP in their mammary glands developed with shorter latency than in wild type mice and metastasized to soft tissues, they did not metastasize to bone (69).

5. SYNGENEIC MODEL OF BREAST TO BONE METASTASIS

As stated above, the most useful model for studying the metastatic spread of breast cancer to bone is one that mimics all steps of the process in humans. This will include spontaneous metastasis from the mammary gland to distant sites, including bone, and a host with an intact immune system.

A model that fulfills these requirements now exists (70). Two cell lines called 4T1.2 and 4T1.13 have a high propensity to metastasize to bone after orthotopic injection into the mammary fat pad (70). They are derived from the 4T1 subline that was originally isolated by Miller and colleagues (71), as an extension of a study in 1978 by Dexter et al. (72) who isolated several distinct lines with differing metastatic capacities from a spontaneous BALB/cfC3H mammary tumor. The isolation of populations of cells with different metastatic properties from a single tumor confirms the heterogeneity of primary mammary tumors.

The 4T1.2 and 4T1.13 clones mimic the clinical disease in that a primary breast tumor grows following orthotopic inoculation into the mammary gland, the cells invade through the stroma into the circulation and colonize distant organs, including lymph nodes, lung and bone. Other sublines isolated by Miller et al. (71) are either non-metastatic (67NR) or weakly metastatic (4T07, 168FARN or 66c14) (Figure 1). Following mammary fat pad inoculation, bone metastases are evident within 25-30 days by histology (Figure 2) and hind leg paralysis is observed in some mice injected with the bone metastasizing clones. This is the first reported mouse model of spontaneous metastasis of breast tumor cells from the primary site in the mammary gland to bone.

The designation of sites of metastasis is shown in Figure 1. These sites were confirmed by detection of overt metastatic nodules using histological techniques and by isolation and growth in culture of drug resistant tumor cells from various organs (70, 71). However, using a more sensitive method for detection of metastases, as described below, we have further refined the sites of metastasis for each of these sublines.

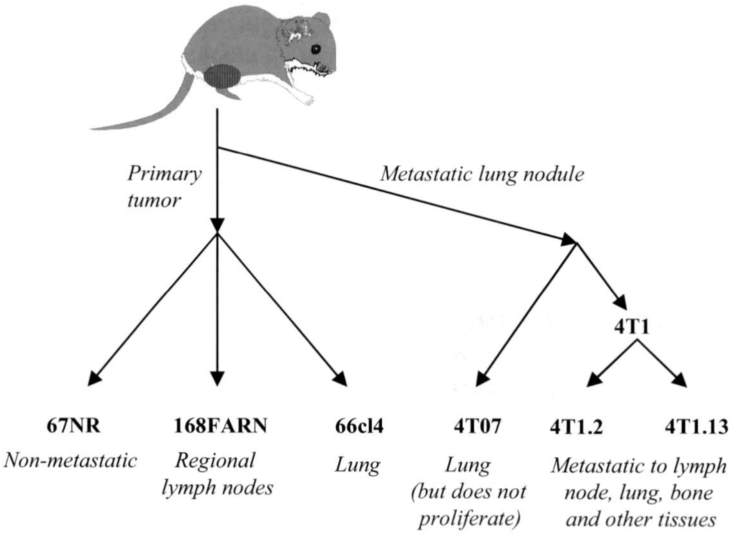

Figure 1. Orthotopic model of breast cancer metastasis to bone. Several tumor sublines have been isolated from a spontaneously arising mammary gland carcinoma. Each subline has a distinct metastatic phenotype. 67NR is non-metastatic, while 168FARN, 66cl4 and 4T07 are weakly metastatic and have a tissue restricted metastatic distribution. 4T1.2 and 4T1.13 are two bone metastasizing tumor clones derived from the lung metastasizing 4T1 subline.

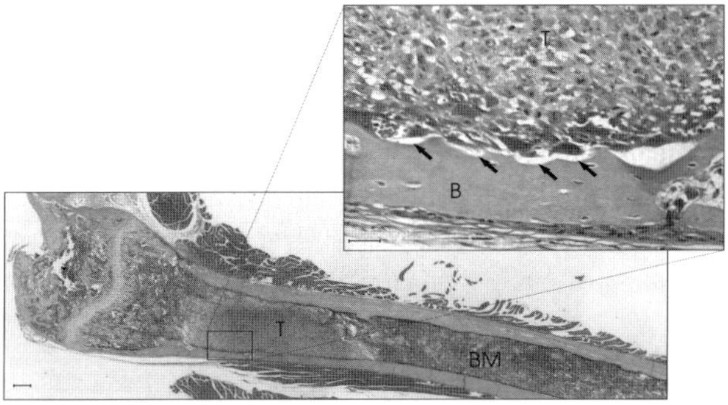

Figure 2. Hematoxylin and eosin staining of a section through the femur of a 4T1.2 tumor bearing mouse, 30 days after inoculation of tumor cells into the mammary gland (x20, scale bar 200mm). At higher magnification (x200, scale bar 25mm), resorption pits (arrows) can be observed in the bone (B) adjacent to the metastatic nodule (T). These pits are not evident in bone adjacent to normal bone marrow (BM).

5.1 Quantitative Measurement of Metastatic Burden

Each tumor line within the model has been tagged with a reporter gene to enable quantitative measurement of tumor burden in different organs by real time PCR. Reporter genes that we have used for this purpose include green fluorescent protein (EGFP), neomycin and puromycin resistance genes. EGFP was abandoned as a reporter gene after it was observed to cause reduced growth and metastasis in mice, presumably due to the EGFP protein acting as an antigen. A similar effect has not been observed with the other two reporter genes. In contrast, EGFP has proven to be a very useful imaging agent for metastases in xenograft models where immune rejection is not an issue (73). Tumor burden has been measured in multiple organs following inoculation of tumor cells into the mammary fat pads of mice (Eckhardt et al., manuscript in preparation). The analysis, reproduced in Figure 3, confirms and further expands the distribution of metastases detected histologically in mice, with the 67NR line failing to metastasize at all, and the other lines metastasizing to varying extents. This method of analysis enables detection of micrometastases not visible by histology. However, when the relative tumor burden increases, there is a good correlation between measurement of tumor burden using this method and by histological assessment (Tavaria et al., submitted for publication).

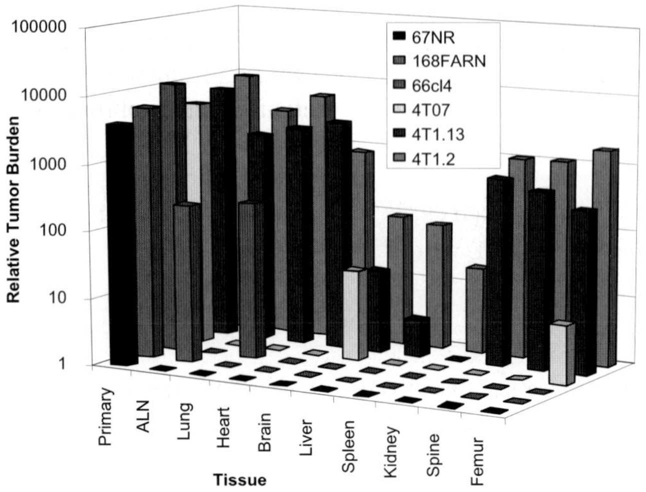

Figure 3. Detection of tumor burden in mouse tissues by real time PCR analysis. Tissue distribution of tumor cells tagged with the neomycin resistance gene following growth of a primary tumor in the mammary fat pad. The relative tumor burden is a measure of the ratio of neomycin positive tumor cells to total cells in the tissue (ALN, axillary lymph node).

5.2 Expression Analysis of the Sublines of the Model

The model is of enormous value for a comparison of the expression profiles of primary tumors with different metastatic capacities, since all sublines are derived from the same spontaneous mammary tumor and are genetically well matched. By cDNA microarray analysis, a number of candidate genes that may have a role in specific metastasis to bone and/or other sites have been found. Using small primary tumors with no necrotic regions (5-7 mm diameter), we have examined the profile of expressed genes using RNA isolated from each tumor. Competitive hybridization to the NIA 15k cDNA array of each metastatic line compared to the non-metastatic 67NR line has generated a number of genes potentially important in metastasis of breast cancer (Eckhardt et al., submitted for publication).

These genes include caveolin-1, which is a regulator of signaling pathways that function through caveolae (74). Loss of caveolin-1 is associated with enhanced metastatic capacity in the murine model and poorer survival in breast cancer patients (Sloan et al., manuscript in preparation). The integrin β3 is another candidate gene for bone metastasis. Increased integrin β3 expression is associated with increased metastasis and enforced expression of this integrin in a poorly metastatic line enhances metastasis, despite causing a reduced growth rate of the primary tumor (Sloan et al., manuscript in preparation). Other interesting candidate genes include protease nexin-1 (a serpin), urokinase plasminogen activator (uPA), a newly described integrin binding protein called nephronectin (75) and a number of ESTs.

5.3 Induced Expression of Genes by Stromal Cells within the Tumor

Whilst the genes mentioned above are differentially expressed in primary tumors with differing metastatic patterns, it is important to recognize that some may be expressed by stromal cells within the tumor rather than by tumor cells. It is now well established that tumor cells exert an influence on the behavior of surrounding normal cells, including vascular endothelial cells, fibroblasts, and cells of the immune system (3, 76). The contribution of these other cell types, including their interaction with the epithelium, requires investigations into the expression profiles of specific cell types. Using this model, specific cell populations from fresh primary tumors of varying metastatic potential and matched metastatic tumors can be immunopurified and analysed independently. Alternatively, laser capture microdissection (LCM) can be used to isolate tumor and stromal cells from frozen tissue. These techniques will potentially be more useful in finding genes important in the stroma and blood vessels, which may be masked when analysing whole tumor preparations. This will also be required in the bone environment to identify the key players in bone resorption, and whether the stroma initiates the tumor production of genes such as PTHrP.

5.4 Therapeutic Applications of the Model

Since the highly metastatic 4T1.2 and 4T1.13 sublines closely mimic aggressive human breast cancer, they allow us to examine the importance of genes found by cDNA microarray analysis in the metastatic process. This can be achieved with relative ease (depending on the gene under study) by using either antisense expression or by stable RNA interference. In addition, induced expression of potential metastasis genes in the less metastatic lines such as 66cl4, may reveal a role for that gene in enhancing metastasis. The mechanism by which each gene functions to promote or suppress metastasis and its potential as a therapeutic target can be determined. The relevance of both novel genes and those previously implicated in the literature, such as PTHrP, can be tested in this model. The quantitative tumor burden assay enables accurate analysis of the impact of the particular gene in metastasis.

It is important to verify that the gene under analysis is relevant to human breast cancer metastasis as well. The development of human tumor tissue arrays has enabled us and other investigators to link expression of a particular gene to clinical outcome for that patient, using a large number of samples arrayed on one slide. If such a correlation is found, the gene becomes a potential target for drug therapy or a useful prognostic marker.

Novel compounds or drugs for which there is some evidence of inhibition of metastasis or tumor growth in bone can be tested in this model with relative ease, again using the relative tumor burden assay as a quantitative measure of drug efficacy.

The development of improved models of breast cancer metastasis to bone and new technologies such as cDNA microarrays and tissue arrays are combining to enable an accurate molecular analysis of this debilitating disease. New molecular targets and specific therapies will be the likely outcomes of these studies.

ACKNOWLEDGEMENTS

The authors would like to thank members of the laboratory, Erica Sloan, Michael Tavaria, Anthony Natoli, Christina Restall, Maria Lelekakis, Kym Stanley, Clare Fritzlaff and Om Narayan for sharing their data. Support from the NIH (CA90291) and the Department of the Army Breast Cancer Research Program (DAMD17-98-1-8144) and DAMD17-01-1-0371 is gratefully acknowledged.

REFERENCES

1. Coleman RE, Rubens RD. The clinical course of bone metastases from breast cancer. Br J Cancer, 55: 61-66, 1987.
2. Klein CA, Blankenstein TJ, Schmidt-Kittler O, Petronio M, Polzer B, Stoecklein NH, Riethmuller G. Genetic heterogeneity of single disseminated tumor cells in minimal residual cancer. Lancet, 360: 683-689, 2002.
3. Wiseman BS, Werb Z. Stromal effects on mammary gland development and breast cancer. Science, 296: 1046-1049, 2002.
4. Chambers AF, Groom AC, MacDonald IC. Dissemination and growth of cancer cells in metastatic sites. Nat Rev Cancer, 2: 563-572, 2002.
5. Liotta LA. An attractive force in metastasis. Nature, 410: 24-25, 2001.
6. Muller A, Homey B, Soto H, Ge N, Catron D, Buchanan ME, McClanahan T, Murphy E, Yuan W, Wagner SN, Barrera JL, Mohar A, Verastegui E, Zlotnik A. Involvement of chemokine receptors in breast cancer metastasis. Nature, 410: 50-56, 2001.
7. Sloan EK, Anderson RL. Genes involved in breast cancer metastasis to bone. Cell Mol Life Sci, 59: 1491-1502, 2002.

8. Parker B, Sukumar S. Distant metastasis in breast cancer: molecular mechanisms and therapeutic targets. Cancer Biol Ther, 2: 14-21, 2003.
9. Chambers AF, MacDonald IC, Schmidt EE, Koop S, Morris VL, Khokha R, Groom, A. C. Steps in tumor metastasis: new concepts from intravital videomicroscopy. Cancer Metastasis Rev, 14: 279-301, 1995.
10. Luzzi KJ, MacDonald IC, Schmidt EE, Kerkvliet N, Morris VL, Chambers AF, Groom, AC. Multistep nature of metastatic inefficiency: dormancy of solitary cells after successful extravasation and limited survival of early micrometastases. Am J Pathol, 153: 865-873, 1998.
11. Mundy GR. Metastasis to bone: causes, consequences and therapeutic opportunities. Nat Rev Cancer, 2: 584-593, 2002.
12. Fedarko NS, Fohr B, Robey PG, Young MF, Fishe LW. Factor H binding to bone sialoprotein and osteopontin enables tumor cell evasion of complement-mediated attack. J Biol Chem, 275: 16666-16672, 2000.
13. Chelouche Lev D, Price JE. Therapeutic intervention with breast cancer metastasis. Crit Rev Eukaryot Gene Expr, 12: 137-150, 2002.
14. Yoneda T, Michigami T, Yi B, Williams PJ, Niewolna M, Hiraga T. Actions of bisphosphonate on bone metastasis in animal models of breast carcinoma. Cancer, 88: 2979-2988, 2000.
15. Body JJ. Effectiveness and cost of bisphosphonate therapy in tumor bone disease. Cancer, 97: 859-865, 2003.
16. Kanis JA. Rationale for the use of bisphosphonates in breast cancer. Acta Oncol, 35 Suppl 5: 61-67, 1996.
17. Body JJ, Bartl R, Burckhardt P, Delmas PD, Diel IJ, Fleisch H, Kanis JA, Kyle RA, Mundy GR, Paterson AH, Rubens RD. Current use of bisphosphonates in oncology. International Bone and Cancer Study Group. J Clin Oncol, 16: 3890-3899, 1998.
18. Diel IJ, Solomayer EF, Costa SD, Gollan C, Goerner R, Wallwiener D, Kaufmann M, Bastert G. Reduction in new metastases in breast cancer with adjuvant clodronate treatment. N Engl J Med, 339: 357-363, 1998.
19. Morony S, Capparelli C, Sarosi I, Lacey DL, Dunstan CR, Kostenuik PJ. Osteoprotegerin inhibits osteolysis and decreases skeletal tumor burden in syngeneic and nude mouse models of experimental bone metastasis. Cancer Res, 61: 4432-4436, 2001.
20. Kostenuik, PJ, Shalhoub V. Osteoprotegerin: a physiological and pharmacological inhibitor of bone resorption. Curr Pharm Des, 7: 613-635, 2001.
21. Reddi AH, Roodman D, Freeman C, Mohla S. Mechanisms of tumor metastasis to the bone: challenges and opportunities. J Bone Miner Res, 18: 190-194, 2003.
22. Boyce BF, Yoneda T, Guise TA. Factors regulating the growth of metastatic cancer in bone. Endocr Relat Cancer, 6: 333-347, 1999.
23. Chirgwin JM, Guise TA. Molecular mechanisms of tumor-bone interactions in osteolytic metastases. Crit Rev Eukaryot Gene Expr, 10: 159-178, 2000.
24. Lacroix M, Siwek B, Marie PJ, Body JJ. Production and regulation of interleukin-11 by breast cancer cells. Cancer Lett, 127: 29-35, 1998.
25. Gillespie MT, Thomas RJ, Pu ZY, Zhou H, Martin TJ, Findlay DM. Calcitonin receptors, bone sialoprotein and osteopontin are expressed in primary breast cancers. Int J Cancer, 73: 812-815, 1997.
26. Johnson RA, Boyce BF, Mundy GR, Roodman GD. Tumors producing human tumor necrosis factor induced hypercalcemia and osteoclastic bone resorption in nude mice. Endocrinology, 124: 1424-1427, 1989.
27. Yin JJ, Selander K, Chirgwin JM, Dallas M, Grubb, BG, Wieser R, Massague J, Mundy GR, Guise TA. TGF-beta signaling blockade inhibits PTHrP secretion by breast cancer cells and bone metastases development. J Clin Invest, 103: 197-206, 1999.

28. Tumber A, Morgan HM, Meikle MC, Hill PA. Human breast-cancer cells stimulate the fusion, migration and resorptive activity of osteoclasts in bone explants. Int J Cancer, 91: 665-672, 2001.
29. Mancino AT, Klimberg VS, Yamamoto M, Manolagas SC, Abe E. Breast cancer increases osteoclastogenesis by secreting M-CSF and upregulating RANKL in stromal cells. J Surg Res, 100: 18-24, 2001.
30. Ishida A, Fujita N, Kitazawa R, Tsuruo,T. Transforming growth factor-beta induces expression of receptor activator of NF-kappa B ligand in vascular endothelial cells derived from bone. J Biol Chem, 277: 26217-26224, 2002.
31. Yi B, Williams PJ, Niewolna M, Wang Y, Yoneda T. Tumor-derived platelet-derived growth factor-BB plays a critical role in osteosclerotic bone metastasis in an animal model of human breast cancer. Cancer Res, 62: 917-923, 2002.
32. Rabbani SA, Xing RH. Role of urokinase (uPA) and its receptor (uPAR) in invasion and metastasis of hormone-dependent malignancies. Int J Oncol, 12: 911-920, 1998.
33. Pecheur I, Peyruchaud O, Serre CM, Guglielmi J, Voland C, Bourre F, Margue C, Cohen-Solal M, Buffet A, Kieffe, N, Clezardin P. Integrin alpha(v)beta3 expression confers on tumor cells a greater propensity to metastasize to bone. FASEB J, 16: 1266-1268, 2002.
34. Maass N, Hojo T, Rosel F, Ikeda T, Jonat W, Nagasaki K. Down regulation of the tumor suppressor gene maspin in breast carcinoma is associated with a higher risk of distant metastasis. Clin Biochem, 34: 303-307, 2001.
35. Lhotak S, Elavathil LJ, Vukmirovic-Popovic S, Duivenvoorden WC, Tozer RG, Singh G. Immunolocalization of matrix metalloproteinases and their inhibitors in clinical specimens of bone metastasis from breast carcinoma. Clin Exp Metastasis, 18: 463-470, 2000.
36. Felding-Habermann B, O'Toole TE, Smith JW, Fransvea E, Ruggeri ZM, Ginsberg MH, Hughes PE, Pampori N, Shattil SJ, Saven A, Mueller BM. Integrin activation controls metastasis in human breast cancer. Proc Natl Acad Sci USA, 98: 1853-1858, 2001.
37. Honore P, Luger NM, Sabino MA, Schwei MJ, Rogers SD, Mach DB, O'Keefe PF, Ramnaraine ML, Clohisy DR, Mantyh PW. Osteoprotegerin blocks bone cancer-induced skeletal destruction, skeletal pain and pain-related neurochemical reorganization of the spinal cord. Nat Med, 6: 521-528, 2000.
38. Shayakhmetov DM, Li ZY, Ni S, Lieber A. Targeting of adenovirus vectors to tumor cells does not enable efficient transduction of breast cancer metastases. Cancer Res, 62: 1063-1068, 2002.
39. Peyruchaud O, Winding B, Pecheur I, Serre CM, Delmas P, Clezardin P. Early detection of bone metastases in a murine model using fluorescent human breast cancer cells: application to the use of the bisphosphonate zoledronic acid in the treatment of osteolytic lesions. J Bone Miner Res, 16: 2027-2034, 2001.
40. Arguello F, Baggs RB, Frantz CN. A murine model of experimental metastasis to bone and bone marrow. Cancer Res, 48: 6876-6881, 1988.
41. Price JE. Metastasis from human breast cancer cell lines. Breast Cancer Res Treat, 39: 93-102, 1996.
42. Teste AM, Sharp JA, Dhanesuan N, Waltham M, Thompson EW. Correlation between extent of osteolytic damage and metastatic burden of human breast cancer metastasis in nude mice: real-time PCR quantitation. Clin Exp Metastasis, 19: 377-383, 2002.
43. Yoneda T, Williams PJ, Hiraga T, Niewolna M, Nishimura RA bone-seeking clone exhibits different biological properties from the MDA-MB-231 parental human breast cancer cells and a brain-seeking clone in vivo and in vitro. J Bone Miner Res, 16: 1486-1495, 2001.
44. Leek RD, Harris AL. Tumor-associated macrophages in breast cancer. J Mammary Gland Biol Neoplasia, 7: 177-189, 2002.

45. Choi SJ, Cruz JC, Craig F, Chung H, Devlin RD, Roodman GD, Alsina M. Macrophage inflammatory protein 1-alpha is a potential osteoclast stimulatory factor in multiple myeloma. Blood, 96: 671-675, 2000.
46. Abe M, Hiura K, Wilde J, Moriyama K, Hashimoto T, Ozaki S, Wakatsuki S, Kosaka M, Kido S, Inoue D, Matsumoto T. Role for macrophage inflammatory protein (MIP)-1alpha and MIP-1beta in the development of osteolytic lesions in multiple myeloma. Blood, 100: 2195-2202, 2002.
47. Warren HS, Smyth MJ. NK cells and apoptosis. Immunol Cell Biol, 77: 64-75, 1999.
48. Smyth MJ, Godfrey DI, Trapani JA. A fresh look at tumor immunosurveillance and immunotherapy. Nat Immunol, 2: 293-299, 2001.
49. Zia A, Schildberg FW, Funke I. MHC class I negative phenotype of disseminated tumor cells in bone marrow is associated with poor survival in R0M0 breast cancer patients. Int J Cancer, 93: 566-570, 2001.
50. Rees RC, Mian S. Selective MHC expression in tumors modulates adaptive and innate antitumor responses. Cancer Immunol Immunother, 48: 374-381, 1999.
51. Zhang GJ, Adachi I. Serum levels of soluble intercellular adhesion molecule-1 and E-selectin in metastatic breast carcinoma: correlations with clinicopathological features and prognosis. Int J Oncol, 14: 71-77, 1999.
52. Cefai D, Favre L, Wattendorf E, Marti A, Jaggi R, Gimmi CD. Role of Fas ligand expression in promoting escape from immune rejection in a spontaneous tumor model. Int J Cancer, 91: 529-537, 2001.
53. Muschen M, Moers C, Warskulat U, Even J, Niederacher D, Beckmann MW. CD95 ligand expression as a mechanism of immune escape in breast cancer. Immunology, 99: 69-77, 2000.
54. Maroulakou IG, Anve M, Garrett L, Green JE. Prostate and mammary adenocarcinoma in transgenic mice carrying a rat C3(1) simian virus 40 large tumor antigen fusion gene. Proc Natl Acad Sci U S A, 91: 11236-11240, 1994.
55. Hennighausen L. Mouse models for breast cancer. Breast Cancer Res, 2: 2-7, 2000.
56. Zhang M, Shi Y, Magit D, Furth PA, Sager R. Reduced mammary tumor progression in WAP-TAg/WAP-maspin bitransgenic mice. Oncogene, 19: 6053-6058, 2000.
57. Sinn E, Muller W, Pattengale P, Tepler I, Wallace R, Leder, P. Coexpression of MMTV/v-Ha-ras and MMTV/c-myc genes in transgenic mice: synergistic action of oncogenes in vivo. Cell, 49: 465-475, 1987.
58. Michaelson JS, Leder P. beta-catenin is a downstream effector of Wnt-mediated tumorigenesis in the mammary gland. Oncogene, 20: 5093-5099, 2001.
59. Deng CX. Tumor formation in Brca1 conditional mutant mice. Environ Mol Mutagen, 39: 171-177, 2002.
60. Guise TA. Parathyroid hormone-related protein and bone metastases. Cancer, 80: 1572-1580, 1997.
61. Suva LJ, Winslow GA, Wettenhall RE, Hammonds RG, Moseley JM, Diefenbach-Jagger H, Rodda CP, Kemp BE, Rodriguez H, Chen EY, et al. A parathyroid hormone-related protein implicated in malignant hypercalcemia: cloning and expression. Science, 237: 893-896, 1987.
62. Moseley JM, Kubota M, Diefenbach-Jagger H, Wettenhall RE, Kemp BE, Suva LJ, Rodda CP, Ebeling PR, Hudson PJ, Zajac JD, et al. Parathyroid hormone-related protein purified from a human lung cancer cell line. Proc Natl Acad Sci USA, 84: 5048-5052, 1987.
63. Rankin W, Grill V, Martin TJ. Parathyroid hormone-related protein and hypercalcemia. Cancer, 80: 1564-1571, 1997.
64. Guise TA, Yin JJ, Thomas RJ, Dallas M, Cui Y, Gillespie MT. Parathyroid hormone-related protein (PTHrP)-(1-139) isoform is efficiently secreted in vitro and enhances breast cancer metastasis to bone in vivo. Bone, 30: 670-676, 2002.

65. Bundred NJ, Ratcliffe WA, Walker RA. Coley S, Morrison JM, Ratcliffe JG. Parathyroid hormone related protein and hypercalcaemia in breast cancer. BMJ, 303: 1506-1509, 1991.
66. Kohno N, Kitazawa S, Sakoda Y, Kanbara Y, Furuya Y, Ohash, O, Kitazawa R. Parathyroid Hormone-related Protein in Breast Cancer Tissues: Relationship between Primary and Metastatic Sites. Breast Cancer, 1: 43-49, 1994.
67. Yoshida A, Nakamura Y, Shimizu A, Harada M, Kameda Y, Nagano A, Inaba M, Asaga T. Significance of the parathyroid hormone-related protein expression in breast carcinoma. Breast Cancer, 7: 215-220, 2000.
68. Henderson M, Danks J, Moseley J, Slavin J, Harris T, McKinlay M, Hopper J, Martin T. Parathyroid hormone-related protein production by breast cancers, improved survival, and reduced bone metastases. J Natl Cancer Inst, 93: 234-237, 2001.
69. Wysolmerski JJ, Dann PR, Zelazny E., Dunbar ME, Insogna KL, Guise TA, Perkins AS. Overexpression of parathyroid hormone-related protein causes hypercalcemia but not bone metastases in a murine model of mammary tumorigenesis. J Bone Miner Res, 17: 1164-1170, 2002.
70. Lelekakis M, Moseley JM, Martin TJ, Hards D, Williams E, Ho P, Lowen D, Javni J, Miller FR, Slavin J, Anderson RL. A novel orthotopic model of breast cancer metastasis to bone. Clin Exp Metastasis, 17: 163-170, 1999.
71. Aslakson CJ, Miller FR. Selective events in the metastatic process defined by analysis of the sequential dissemination of subpopulations of a mouse mammary tumor. Cancer Res, 52: 1399-1405, 1992.
72. Dexter DL, Kowalski HM, Blazar BA, Fligiel Z, Vogel R, Heppner GH. Heterogeneity of tumor cells from a single mouse mammary tumor. Cancer Res, 38: 3174-3181, 1978.
73. Li X, Wang J, An Z, Yang M, Baranov E, Jiang P, Sun F, Moossa AR, Hoffman RM. Optically imageable metastatic model of human breast cancer. Clin Exp Metastasis, 19: 347-350, 2002.
74. Lee SW, Reimer CL, Oh P, Campbell DB, Schnitzer JE. Tumor cell growth inhibition by caveolin re-expression in human breast cancer cells. Oncogene, 16: 1391-1397, 1998.
75. Brandenberger R, Schmidt A, Linton J, Wang D, Backus C, Denda S, Muller U, Reichardt LF. Identification and characterization of a novel extracellular matrix protein nephronectin that is associated with integrin alpha8beta1 in the embryonic kidney. J Cell Biol, 154: 447-458, 2001.
76. Liotta LA, Kohn EC. The microenvironment of the tumor-host interface. Nature, 411: 375-379, 2001.

Chapter 2

QUANTITATION OF BONE METASTASIS IN EXPERIMENTAL SYSTEMS

Julie A. Sharp[1] and Erik W. Thompson[1, 2,]
[1]*Department of Surgery, University of Melbourne, St. Vincent's Institute of Medical Research, and* [2]*Bernard O'Brien Institute of Microsurgery, St. Vincent's Hospital, Fitzroy, Australia*

1. INTRODUCTION

Animal models are important tools to investigate the pathogenesis and develop treatment strategies for bone metastases in humans. However, there are few spontaneous models of bone metastasis despite the fact that rodents (rats and mice) and other animals (dogs and cats) often spontaneously develop cancer. Therefore, most experimental models of bone metastasis in rodents require injection or implantation of neoplastic cells into orthotopic locations, bones, or the left ventricle of the heart.

2. METASTATIC BONE DISEASE

Bone is a frequent site of metastases of the most common tumors, e.g., breast carcinoma and prostate carcinoma. The functions of the skeleton, calcium homeostasis and mechanical support, are carried out by the continuous destruction and rebuilding of bone, a process known as bone remodeling. Multinucleated, hemopoietically derived osteoclasts, which are related to macrophages, digest the bone, and mesenchymal-derived osteoblasts rebuild it. This is kept in balance by finely regulated processes whereby osteoblast lineage cells respond to homeostatic signals and release factors that regulate osteoclast generation and activity. Cells that participate in inflammation and immunity also can stimulate osteoclast formation and

G. Singh and W. Orr (eds.), Bone Metastasis and Molecular Mechanisms, 19-30.

lead to bone destruction. Tumor cells most likely interfere with these physiologic processes, seeding within the bone and establishing metastases. Bone metastases from breast carcinoma are generally associated with bone destruction which occurs in response to factors secreted by metastatic cells. Some of these factors secreted by the metastatic cells activate osteoclasts, although in some cases others are proteases that degrade bone collagen. In contrast, the balance is altered in prostate carcinoma bone metastases, which are predominantly osteosclerotic.

2.1 Animal Models

Injection of cancer cell lines into the left cardiac ventricle of immunodeficient mice is a widely used animal model of bone/bone marrow metastasis. This experimental setting closely resembles the clinical situation of minimal residual disease after removal of the primary tumor. However, detection of bone metastasis by radiography makes it a less-than-ideal model of minimal residual disease. In fact, radiologically evident osteolytic/osteosclerotic metastases are a late and macroscopic event in the evolution of metastatic bone disease. Thus, the model lacks the sensitivity that would be necessary to dissect the initial processes, such as the "angiogenic switch," essential for tumor progression. Furthermore, the radiological detection of osteolytic and/or osteosclerotic metastases is an indirect measure of the tumor burden. Only a parallel histomorphometric analysis allows the distinction between a therapeutic effect exerted directly on tumor cells or indirectly through inhibition of bone resorption. Therefore, more sensitive methods to detect and monitor directly metastatic growth in bone marrow/bone of whole animals need to be developed.

2.1.1 The MDA-MB-231 Breast Cancer Model

Since bone metastasis occurs very rarely from current spontaneous or experimental metastasis models of carcinoma cells in immunocompromised mice, an arterial seeding model involving the direct intracardiac injection of the cells into the left ventricle has been developed to mimic the process of metastasis (1, 2). This model has also been used for orthotopic injection into the mammary fat pad and tibia. The breast cancer cell line MDA-MB-231 has been widely used as a working model for *in vivo* metastatic studies in immunocompromised mice. MDA-MB-231 cells have a high propensity to metastasize to bone and soft organs when injected intracardially, grow well as xenographs, metastasize to the lymph nodes and lungs from the mammary fat pad, and grow well within the bone environment of the tibia. For these reasons this model offers a great medium to study many aspects of cancer metastasis and treatment.

3. QUANTITATION IS A KEY ISSUE

3.1 Bone Damage

Bone destruction can be monitored by X-ray, mammography, Faxitron or phase contrast imaging, all which allows visualization of the degree of bone degradation caused by the metastatic tumor. Histomorphometry techniques can be used to provide more information about tumor/bone interactions and impact the tumor has on the bone environment.

In some cases, metastases can be osteoblastic which is a result of factors secreted by the tumor cells influencing the osteoblasts and results in increased bone density and bone deposits. These types of lesions can also be monitored by these techniques.

3.1.1 Histomorphometry and Animal Models of Metastasis

Bone histomorphometry provides quantitative information about bone mass, architecture and turnover. Undecalcified sections are prepared using methyl methacrylate embedding and decalcified sections with paraffin or glycol methacrylate. A variety of histochemical and immunohistochemical stains can be performed to measure cellular counts of osetoblasts and osteoclasts, mineralizing surface, mineral absorption rate, bone formation rate, bone porosity, bone volume, osteoid surface (volume and thickness) and proliferation rates of tumor cells.

In experimental models of bone metastasis, there is evidence that osteolysis and colonisation of the bone marrow by the tumor can be reduced by strategies that inhibit the release or production of proteases (3, 4) or by overexpressing tissue inhibitors of matrix metalloproteinases in metastatic cells (2). The matrix metalloproteinases are mediators of homeostatic bone growth and remodeling (5) and are likely to contribute to the invasion and metastasis of malignant tumors in bone (6, 7). On this basis, Lee et al. (8) have postulated and shown that a synthetic inhibitor of matrix metalloproteinases, Batimastat (BB-94), inhibits the activity of matrix metalloproteinases expressed by MDA-MB-231 human breast carcinoma cells, and blocks the ability of these cells to degrade osteoblast-like matrices or to form resorption pits in cortical bone. *In vivo*, where more than one cell type may be involved in bone destruction, treatment of tumor-bearing animals with Batimastat inhibited tumor-associated osteolysis, tumor growth, and the replacement of marrow by tumor. By using histomorphometry to analyse the metastatic lesions, the ability to distinguish between osteolysis, tumor burden, and marrow replacement was achieved which can not be accomplished by more conventional radiological measurements. The effects of Batimastat treatment on the formation of bone metastases by MDA-MB-231 cells were striking. The marked osteolytic effects of the tumor were blocked in both femoral and vertebral bone, accompanied by diminished extension of tumor into the medullary long bone, decreased tumor volume, sparing of haematopoietic tissue, and a decrease in the number of metastases found in the vertebral bodies. Winding et al. (9) also found considerable inhibition of bone metastasis in the MDA-MB-231-B (bone-metastasis selected) model using either Batimastat or Galardin (GM-6001, another broad-spectrum MMP-inhibitor), and in fact were able to reverse established bone damage. These lesions were also assessed radiologically with morphometric analysis. Our own group has found similar retardation of the onset of osteolytic metastasis monitored with weekly Faxitron, using the gelatinase-selective MMP inhibitor Prinomastat [AG 3340; Agouron-Pfizer, (10)].

3.2 Tumor Burden

Quantitation of tumor burden has been demonstrated in numerous ways using essentially the same technique. Quantitative real time PCR provides an accurate and sensitive modality for detection of tumor cells by amplifications of a given sequence that is unique to the cells employed. These sequences include the bacterially derived B-galactosidase (Lac-Z) and neomycin resistance genes, the luciferase gene and the gene encoding green fluorescent protein (GFP), all which have been genetically introduced into cancer cell lines to identify and quantitate the metastatic cells within the host rodent model organism. Another method recently being used employs the detection of human specific Alu sequences that are a normal component of the human genome to identify and quantitate the metastatic human cells within the host organism.

3.2.1 Quantitation of *in vivo* Breast Cancer Models

We employ the human breast cancer cell line MDA-MB-231 transduced with a bacterially derived Lac Z sequence (MDA-MB-231-BAG) as a model of breast cancer metastasis. A sensitive quantitative real-time polymerase chain reaction (PCR) method that amplifies the genomically incorporated Lac Z sequence in the MDA-MB-231-BAG cells is used to detect and quantitate bone and soft organ metastasis in nude mice intracardially inoculated with these cells. Amplification of this sequence enables us to specifically detect these cells in mouse organs and bones. PCR detection was linear, specific, more sensitive than conventional PCR, and could be used to directly quantitate metastatic burden in bone and soft organs. Attesting to the sensitivity and specificity of the PCR detection strategy, as few as several hundred metastatic MDA-MB-231 cells were detectable in 100 micron segments of paraffin-embedded lung tissue, and only in samples adjacent to sections that scored positive by histological detection (Figure 1). Moreover, the measured real-time PCR metastatic burden in the bone environment displayed a high correlation to the degree of osteolytic damage observed by high resolution X-ray analysis (Figure 2). Such a direct linear relationship to tumor burden and bone damage substantiates the so-called 'vicious cycle' hypothesis in which metastatic tumor cells promote the release of factors from the bone which continue to stimulate the tumor cells. The model provides a useful tool for molecular and cellular analysis of human breast cancer metastasis to bone and soft organs, can easily be extended to other cell /marker /organ systems, and should also find application in preclinical assessment of anti-metastatic modalities (11).

A similar model has also been used for detection of a murine mammary adenocarcinoma cell line (Clone 66) transduced with neomycin resistance gene injected orthotopically into immunocompromised mice for detection of cells within bone marrow. PCR for the neomycin gene performed on bone marrow cells harvested from tumor bearing mice demonstrated as few as 10^2 injected tumor cells produced bone marrow micrometastases at 4 weeks postinjection. Small foci of tumor cells were identified in the mammary fatpad without gross evidence of primary tumors. Higher doses of tumor cells produced bone marrow micrometastases, detectable by PCR, at one week post-injection. Constructs containing GFP and the neomycin resistance gene were also transduced into Clone 66 cells (Cl66-GFPneo) and injected into the mammary fat pad. GFP transduced tumor cells were identified in multiple tissues in addition to bone marrow by flow cytometric analysis (FACS) but less than 13% of the animals developed gross metastases. This model is a clinically relevant tool for the analysis of organ specificity of metastasis (12).

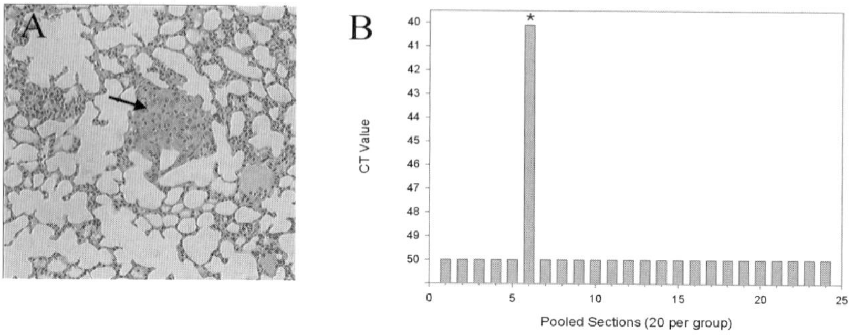

Figure 1. Analysis of micrometastases in mice lungs by real-time PCR and histology. Animals were inoculated with MDA-MB-231 BAG cells into the mammary fat pad. After 45-55 days the mice were sacrificed, the lungs removed, and any micrometastases analyzed by histology and real-time PCR. A) Haematoxlyin and eosin stained section of mice lung tissue showing micrometastasis (arrowed). B) Real-time PCR of DNA extracted from a series of paraffin embedded sections across the entire lung. Each group represents 20 pooled sections within the series. The asterisk corresponds to the group of sections represented by A.
This figure is reprinted from Clinical Experimetal Metastasis Vol. 19(5): 377-383, Figure 4, Copyright 2002 with kind permission of Kluwer Academic Publishers.

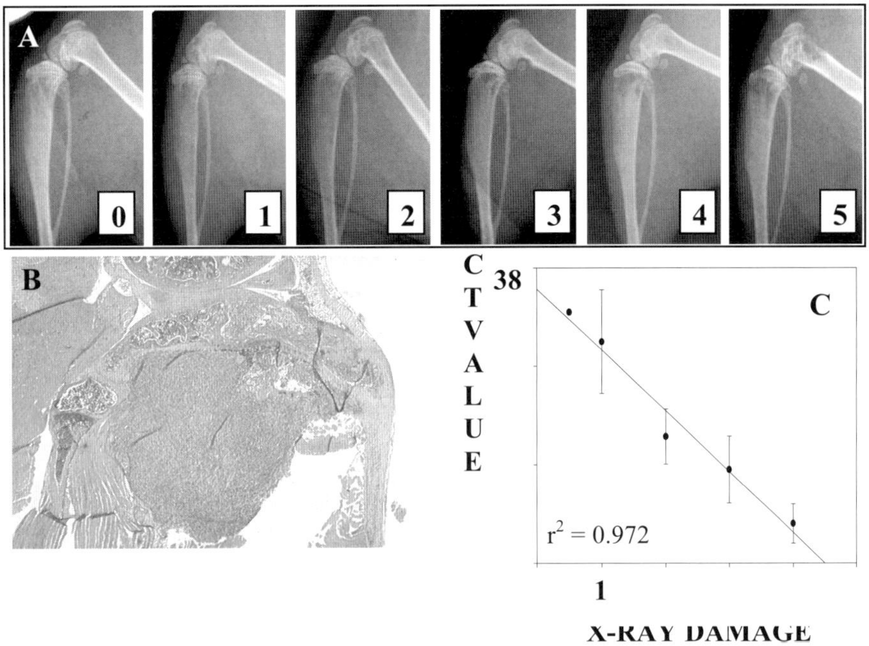

Figure 2. Comparison of the metastatic burden in bone and the degree of osteolytic damage observed. The long bones from mice following intracardiac inoculation of MDA-MB-231 BAG cells were analyzed by high resolution X-ray analysis and by real-time PCR. The degree of osteolytic damage was scored on a semi-quantitative scale, with a score of 0 representing no visible damage and a score of 5 representing severe damage. Examples are illustrated in panel (A), and a haematoxlyin and eosin stained section of tumor growth in the tibia region for a damage 'rating 4' is given in panel (B). There was a direct correlation between the severity of osteolytic damage observed and the metastatic burden in bone detected by real-time PCR (expressed as CT value) panel (C). The error bars represent the range of the number of cancer cells detected within the different damage scales. This figure is reprinted from Clinical Experimetal Metastasis Vol. 19(5): 377-383, Figure 5, Copyright 2002 with kind permission of Kluwer Academic Publishers.

3.2.2 Pain

Bone cancer pain is very common, and this type of pain can be extremely debilitating. Development of an experimental model for studying this condition is critical to advancing an understanding of the mechanisms that cause pain in patients with malignant disease.

A murine model of bone cancer has been used to combine the extent of tumor-induced bone destruction, pain, and neurochemical characterization of the peripheral and central nervous systems in order to investigate bone cancer pain. Disease-induced bone destruction was assessed by radiographs and histomorphometry. Pain was assessed by spontaneous and elicited behaviors, and neurochemical analysis involved immunohistochemical detection of hyperalgesic peptides and neurochemical markers.

Mice with distal femoral sarcomas exhibited behavioral and neurochemical measures of pain. The pain condition created by malignant bone disease was distinct neurochemically from inflammatory and neuropathic pain states. Experimental evidence indicated that both disease-induced osteolysis and tumors themselves contributed to the generation of pain and that peripheral and central sensitization of the nervous system was present (13). Interestingly, one of the major benefits of bisphosphonates, which retard osteolytic destruction of bone and are used clinically in breast and prostate cancer, is pain reduction.

3.2.3 Real Time Imaging

The development of new anticancer strategies requires more sensitive and less invasive methods to detect and monitor *in vivo* minimal residual disease in cancer models. Improvements in the imaging of experimental animals *in vivo* using fluorescent markers or light emitted from luciferase have led to increased sensitivity of detection and more accurate quantification of bone metastases which can be detected externally by sensitive detection systems. Cancer cell lines permanently transfected either with the firefly luciferase (*Luc*) or GFP have been used to monitor local tumor growth (14) and development of metastasis to different organs in living mice (15). Clinical and experimental observations indicate that the hematopoietic marrow, rather than the bone tissue, is the initial site of cancer cell seeding. Indeed, small clusters of cancer cells (micrometastases) can be detected in a vast proportion of the bone marrow aspirates of patients affected by a variety of epithelial cancers with no radiological or scintigraphic evidence of bone metastasis at the time of diagnosis and/or surgery of the primary tumor (16). Micrometastases represent the pathophysiological basis of minimal residual disease (17-19) that will eventually lead to cancer relapse as overt metastases. However, they cannot be detected by conventional staging methods and are poorly influenced by current treatment (19). Hence, there is a need for alternative therapeutic strategies that should be tested in experimental models able to mimic micrometastatic spread.

For example, imaging of human prostate carcinoma PC-3M cells transfected with luciferase, following injection into the left ventricle, has demonstrated that there is rapid localization of tumor cells to bones and other organs, such as the kidneys and lungs. Wetterwald et al. (20) have demonstrated that whole-body bioluminescent reporter imaging (BRI) effectively allows sensitive localization and growth monitoring of minimal metastatic deposits in the bone marrow at a stage largely preceding tumor-induced osteolysis.

3.3 Prostate Cancer Models

Prostate cancer metastasis has two defining clinical characteristics: a tendency to involve bone and a marked osteosclerotic response of the bone to the presence of metastatic cells. Prostate cancer bone metastasis causes tremendous morbidity, including pain, impaired mobility, pathologic fractures, spinal cord compression, and other problems. Gross, clinically significant, metastatic deposits develop in bone long before metastases to soft viscera become apparent (21-23). The marked increase in the turnover of bone matrix associated with the presence of prostate cancer cells in bone is often recognized as an osteosclerotic response on radiographic imaging studies. It is well accepted, however, that both bone formation and bone breakdown are present within metastatic deposits (24-26).

Nemeth et al. (27) described the SCID (severe combined immunodeficient)–human model of prostate cancer metastasis, in which a variety of human and mouse organ environments were implanted into SCID mice to serve as a target for human prostate cancer cells. They found that a variety of human prostate cancer cell types preferred to form tumors in the human bone environment than in other human or mouse organ environments. They also demonstrated a bone response ranging from mostly osteolytic to mostly osteoblastic, depending on the type of prostate cancer cells introduced into the bone. Bone tumors formed by the PC3 prostate cancer cell line were consistently osteolytic in nature, suggesting that this model could be used to study the degradative portion of the bone turnover cycle. Tumors developed in the human bone cavity but not in the mouse skeleton. A similar system involving non-obese diabetic (NOD)/SCID mice implanted with adult human bone fragments has also been described recently (28). While these models can be used to explore prostate cancer growth potential in bone, they are not useful for exploring the metastatic events that result in tumor cells establishing in the bone environment. Tumor cells can colonize the human bone fragment after either intravenous injection or direct injection into the bone fragment but not after growth of a primary tumor. The models do, however, avoid the incompatibility issue of human tumor cells in murine stromal tissue. A final point that distinguishes the few existing prostate cancer models from the real disease is the fact that PC3 and DU-145 tumors are osteolytic, whereas those of LnCaP are both osteolytic and osteoblastic (27). The metastases of human prostate cancer are predominantly osteoblastic or mixed blastic and lytic.

17. Hirsch-Ginsberg C. Detection of minimal residual disease: relevance for diagnosis and treatment of human malignancies. Annu Rev Med, 49: 111-122, 1998.
18. Kostle WJ, Brodowicz T, Hejna M, Wiltschke C, Zielinski CC. Detection of minimal residual disease in patients with cancer: a review of techniques, clinical implications, and emerging therapeutic consequences. Cancer Detect Prev, 24: 376-403, 2000.
19. Klein CA. The biology and analysis of single disseminated tumor cells. Trends Cell Biol, 10: 489-493, 2000.
20. Wetterwald A, van der Pluijm G, Que I, Sijmons B, Buijs J, Karperien M, Lowik CW, Gautschi E, Thalmann GN, Cecchini MG. Optical imaging of cancer metastasis to bone marrow: a mouse model of minimal residual disease. Am J Pathol, 160: 1143-1153, 2002.
21. Glaves D. Mechanisms of metastasis: prostate cancer. Prog Clin Biol Res, 239: 329-345, 1987.
22. Saitoh H, Hida M, Shimbo T, Nakamura K, Yamagata J, Satoh T. Metastatic patterns of prostatic cancer. Correlation between sites and number of organs involved. Cancer, 54: 3078-3084, 1984.
23. Bubendorf L, Schopfer A, Wagner U, Sauter G, Moch H, Willi N, Gasser TC, Mihatsch, MJ. Metastatic patterns of prostate cancer: an autopsy study of 1,589 patients. Hum Pathol, 31: 578-583, 2000.
24. Revilla M, Arribas I, Sanchez-Chapado M, Villa LF, Bethencourt F, Rico H. Total and regional bone mass and biochemical markers of bone remodeling in metastatic prostate cancer. Prostate, 35: 243-247, 1998.
25. Akimoto S, Furuya Y, Akakura K, Ito H. Comparison of markers of bone formation and resorption in prostate cancer patients to predict bone metastasis. Endocr J, 45: 97-104, 1998.
26. Takeuchi S, Arai K, Saitoh H, Yoshida, K, Miura M. Urinary pyridinoline and deoxypyridinoline as potential markers of bone metastasis in patients with prostate cancer. J Urol, 156: 1691-1695, 1996.
27. Nemeth JA, Harb JF, Barroso U Jr, He Z, Grignon DJ, Cher ML. Severe combined immunodeficient-hu model of human prostate cancer metastasis to human bone. Cancer Res, 59: 1987-1993, 1999.
28. Yonou H, Yokose T, Kamijo T, Kanomata N, Hasebe T, Nagai K, Hatano T, Ogawa Y, Ochiai A. Establishment of a novel species- and tissue-specific metastasis model of human prostate cancer in humanized non-obese diabetic/severe combined immunodeficient mice engrafted with human adult lung and bone. Cancer Res, 61: 2177-2182, 2001.
29. Thompson TC, Park SH, Timme TL, Ren C, Eastham JA, Donehower LA, Bradley A, Kadmon D, Yang G. Loss of p53 function leads to metastasis in ras+myc-initiated mouse prostate cancer. Oncogene, 10: 869-879, 1995.
30. Rosol TJ, Tannehill-Gregg SH, LeRoy BE, Mandl S, Contag CH. Animal models of bone metastasis. Cancer, 97: 748-757, 2003.

Chapter 3

COMPARATIVE MORPHOMETRIC STUDY ON BONE REMODELING IN HUMAN SPECIMENS AND IN EXPERIMENTAL MODELS OF METASTATIC BONE DISEASE

Snezana Vukmirovic-Popovic, Eric Seidlitz, F. William Orr*, and Gurmit Singh
Juravinski Cancer Centre, Mc Master University, Hamilton Ontario, Canada
**Department of Pathology, University of Manitoba, Winnipeg, Manitoba, Canada*

Metastatic cancer is the most common malignant tumor affecting bone and is accompanied by significant clinical morbidity, including pain, osteolysis, pathological fracture, spinal compression syndromes and hypercalcemia. Bone destruction is a marked clinical feature and the major source of morbidity associated with bone metastases. Most of these clinical features can be related to structural changes in bone that are caused by effects of the tumor on normal processes of bone remodeling.

1. QUALITATIVE HISTOLOGICAL OBSERVATIONS IN CLINICAL SAMPLES

During physiological bone remodeling, bone resorption by osteoclasts is closely coupled to bone formation by osteoblasts to maintain dynamic homeostasis. Once cancer colonizes bone, tumors can cause two distinct but overlapping types of skeletal lesions (i.e., osteolytic and osteoblastic) (1, 2, 3). In malignant osteolysis, a response often seen in breast cancer, the coupling process is dysregulated showing dramatic increases in bone resorption, impaired secondary osteoblast responses, and a net bone deficit

G. Singh and W. Orr (eds.), Bone Metastasis and Molecular Mechanisms, 31-48.

(1, 4, 5). In prostate cancer, the presence of tumor cells in the bone often changes osteoblastic activity, resulting in reduced formation of normal lamellar bone, increased formation of abnormal woven bone, and net bone overproduction (6). To some extent there is almost always bone formation on a microscopic level in osteolytic bone metastasis, even if it can not be detected by standard imaging modalities (1). There are quantitative differences in osteoclastic bone resorption between breast carcinoma and the other types of metastatic carcinoma, such as renal and sqamous cell carcinoma (7, 8).

It is generally accepted that trabecular bone strength depends not only on bone volume but also on its structure (9, 10). Bone fractures are one of the most important complications and a main source of morbidity in patients with bone metastasis. Breast cancer is the most common cause of pathological fractures. (5, 11). Because malignancy-associated focal bone loss at sites of tumor osteolysis produces different clinical manifestations (e.g., fracture/no fracture), it is likely that the pathophysiologies of these processes differ. For example, our previous comparison of patients with and without pathological fractures revealed differences in bone remodeling judged by histomorphometry and microstructural examination. Furthermore, node-strut analysis showed increased disconnectivity and decreased connectivity suggesting more pronounced microstructural changes in the fracture group compared to the non-fracture (12) group. Bone fracture can also be a manifestation of metastatic prostate carcinoma (13). Reduced formation of normal lamellar bone and production of woven bone which is less strong than lamellar bone might contribute to bone strength and fracture risk.

1.1 Histological Patterns in Human Bone Biopsies

The most commonly encountered microscopic bone reaction in metastatic breast cancer is a mixed picture of both osteolysis and osteosclerosis (1). Our study on bone biopsies from patients with metastatic breast carcinoma revealed varying degrees of morphological changes related to bone resorption and bone formation. Osteoclast numbers, lacunar osteolysis, and trabecular fragmentation varied from case to case. Bone trabeculae were surrounded by sheets of malignant cells with tubule formations or solid cell clusters, with varying amounts of fibrovascular stroma. Morphological findings of bone formation included different presentations such as onion-like sclerosis layers on inactive bone surface, spongy sclerosis on active bone surfaces and networks of primitive woven bone in fibrovascular stroma (Figure 1a, b). Different histological findings were observed in the occult metastasis compared to the symptomatic bone metastasis with radiologically detectable bone lesions. Although, histologically a large part of the bone marrow was replaced by metastatic tumor, extensive osteolysis or osteoclastic bone resorption was not observed. There was also evidence of new bone formation rising from the quiescent bone surfaces (Figure 1c, d).

Osteosclerosis is the next most common predominating bone reaction, often seen in prostate cancer and less common in lung cancer (1). Prostate cancer metastases are predominantly osteosclerotic, but woven bone formation is accompanied by progressive lamellar bone destruction. Areas of erosions are also seen on the surface of bony trabeculae in regions free of tumor. The analysis of human bone specimens in polarized light reveals osteoclastic bone resorption of lamellar bone replaced by new abnormal woven bone producing the well-recognized bone forming metastasis (14).

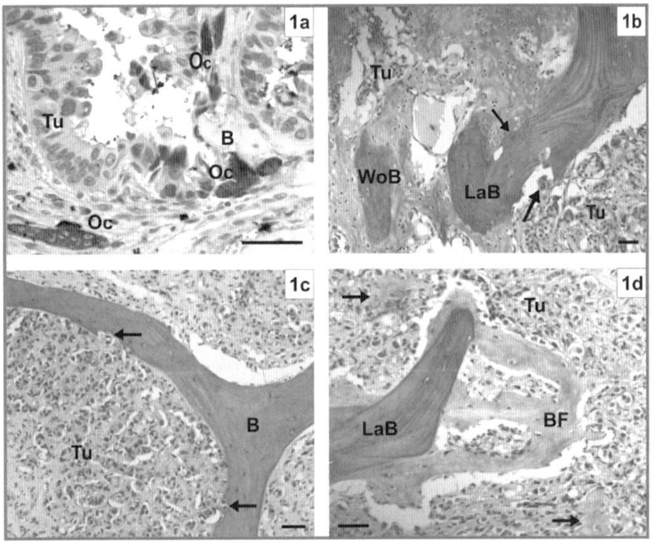

Figure 1 Representative histological findings in bone metastases. Femoral bone biopsies from patient with metastatic breast carcinoma.

(a) Osteolytic bone metastasis. TRAP-positive osteoclasts on the bone surface and in the tumour tissue surrounding the bone trabecula (original magnification x400; TRAP staining).

(b) Reactive new bone formation on one side of a lamellar bone trabecula (thin arrow), with osteoclast-mediated bone resorption on the opposite side of the trabecula (thick arrow). New stromal woven bone formation with irregular orientation of collagen fibers in contrast to the regular orientation in lamellar bone (original magnification x100; H&E staining, polarized light).

(c) Occult bone metastasis with rarely observed microresorptions (arrows) along bone trabeculae (original magnification x400, H&E staining).

(d) Occult bone metastasis showing de novo bone formation on quiescent bone surfaces and in tumour stroma (arrows) (original magnification x400, H&E staining, polarized light).

The rarely reported intertrabecular type of metastasis is characterized by an infiltration of tumor cells into the bone marrow space without a significant alteration of the trabecular bone and no visible lesions by radiology (2, 15, 16). Radiologically undetectable metastatic lesions have been documented as "occult bone metastasis" (17). Some oncologists differentiate bone metastasis with bone destruction from bone marrow metastasis with no bone destruction (18). The mechanism underlying the development and changes in bone remodeling of this type of metastases has not been extensively examined. Based on our recent study using bone histomorphometry and node-strut analysis, occult metastasis represents a separate subtype of metastasis compared to the symptomatic bone metastasis (12).

2. EXPERIMENTAL MODELS OF BONE METASTASIS

Several tumor models have been used to study bone metastasis experimentally. Intracardiac injection has been widely employed as a means to obtain bone colonization by established non-human tumor cell lines in immunocompetent animals or human cancer cell lines in immunodeficient animals (19, 20, 21). Animal models of bone metastasis can provide excellent information about tumor-bone interactions and the mechanisms of action of tumor cells during bone colonization at the tissue level. For example, the estrogen-independent human breast cancer cell line, MDA-MB-231 cells is widely accepted as a suitable model to study osteolytic bone metastasis (22, 23). Unfortunately, osteosclerotic type of prostate cancer metastasis to bone has been difficult to mimic in animal models. Osteolysis is the predominant metastatic phenotype in animals injected with prostate cancer cells (e.g., PC-3, LNCap, PA III) (20, 24, 25).

The syngeneic Dunning MAT-LyLu rate prostate cancer model has been argued to be the first described primarily osteoblastic model (26). Human, estrogen dependent breast carcinoma cells, MCF-7 have also been reported to develop osteosclerotic bone metastases after initial bone resorption (21). However, the bone formation capacity of estrogen-dependant human breast cancer cells (e.g., MCF-7 and T-47D) is still not clear since, in order to support the growth of these breast cancer cells, it is necessary to give supplementation of estrogen because there are insufficient levels of estrogen in female nude mice. It is possible that the administration of estrogen in this model could stimulate bone formation, leading to misinterpretation of the model as osteoblastic bone metastatic model (20).

2.1 Qualitative Histological Observations

Using previously described procedures (19, 26, 27, 28), we have studied the morphological and morphometric alterations of bone remodeling in three animal models of bone metastases. First, the MDA-MB-231 tumor in female nude mice (BALB/c nu/nu) has been found to be a hypercellular tumor that causes an osteoclastic bone resorbing response four weeks after cell injection. A stromal host bone response, commonly seen in human bone metastasis, was not present (Figure 2a, b, c). Second, the murine melanoma B16/F1 tumor in C57BL/6 female mice has been found to be a very aggressive tumor with extensive tumor necrosis and massive bone cell colonization 12 days after cell injection, forming osteolytic bone metastases (Figure 2). The Mat-LyLu tumor, forming bone metastases approximately 12 days after cell inoculation in male Copenhagen rats, causes osteolytic femoral bone metastases, associated with extensive tumor necrosis and osteoclastic-mediated bone resorption. However, spinal bone metastases in this tumor were of a mixed osteoblastic-osteolytic type. Stromal new bone formation as a result of intramembranous ossification was associated with development of a fibrous stroma in the host bone (Figure 3). Reactive new woven bone formation, arising from quiescent bone surfaces, was also noted. Subperiosteal colonization was present in both MDA-MB-231 and MAT-LyLu *in vivo* models (Figure 2c, f). Subperiosteal tumor metastasis is a typical metastatic site in animal experimental models that is not often present in human bone metastasis. It has been previously explained by tumor cell colonization based on anatomical arterial microvascularization of animal bone (20). Subperiosteal tumor localization can produce extensive cortical bone metastasis leading to cortical perforation. Bone metastasis from lung cancer is the only described human periosteal metastasis (20). Human skeletal metastases are most often intramedullary and typically involve the cortex only in the advanced phase of metastatic bone disease (7).

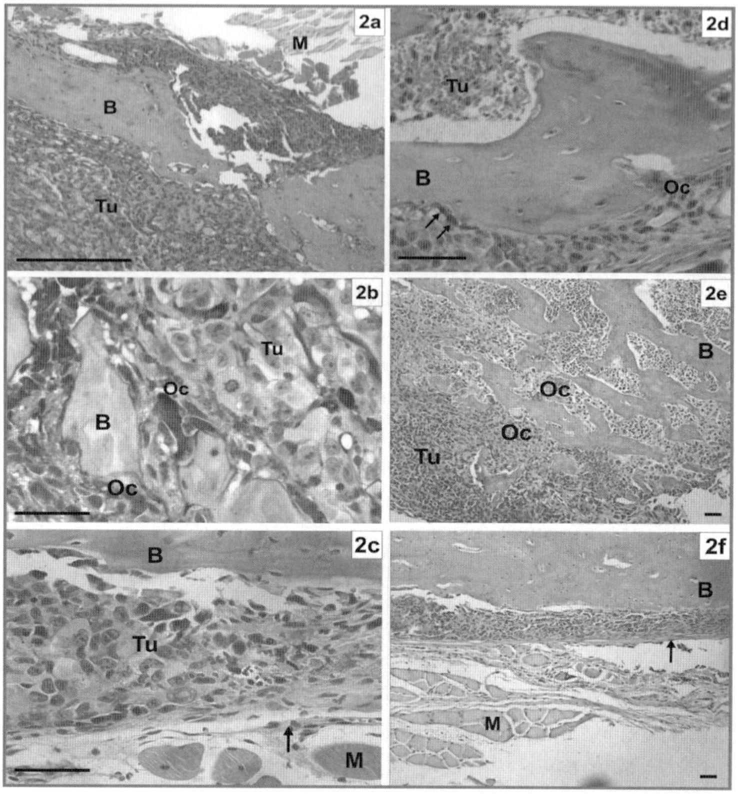

Figure 2. Animal models of osteolytic femoral bone metastasis.

(a) MDA-MB-231 breast cancer metastasis with extensive marrow colonization and cortical perforation invading into the surrounding muscle tissue (original magnification x400, H&E staining).

(b) MDA-MB-231 breast cancer metastasis with numerous TRAP-positive osteoclasts on the bone surface and in the tumour tissue (original magnification x400; TRAP staining).

(c) Subperiosteal MDA-MB-231 cell colonization involving the space between the cortex and periosteum (arrow) (original magnification x400; H&E staining).

(d) B16/F1 melanoma osteolytic femoral bone metastasis with extensive zones of tumour necrosis, numerous pigmented tumour cells on bone surface (arrows) and osteoclastic bone resorption (original magnification x400, H&E staining).

(e) MAT-LyLu osteolytic femoral bone metastasis with osteoclastic bone resorption and extensive tumour necrosis (original magnification x400, H&E staining).

(f) Subperiosteal MAT-LyLu cell colonization involving the space between the cortex and periosteum (arrow) (original magnification x100, H&E staining).

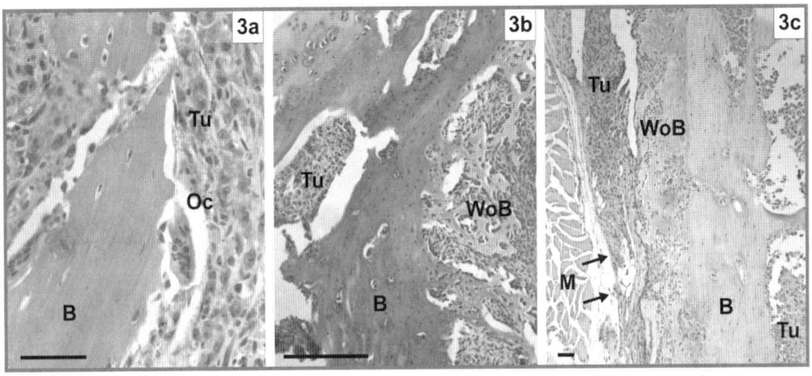

Figure 3. MAT-LyLu mixed type of spinal bone metastasis showing osteolysis and osteosclerosis.
(a) Osteoclastic bone resorption (original magnification x400, H&E staining).
(b) Reactive new woven bone formation (original magnification x400, H&E staining).
(c) Subperiosteal new woven bone formation (original magnification x100, H&E staining, polarized light).

A comparative example of breast carcinoma from clinical samples and in a corresponding animal model is shown in Figure 4. Human breast carcinoma often consisted of abundant fibrous stroma in metastatic bone lesions. Stromal new bone formation as a result of intramembranous ossification was associated with development of a fibrous stroma (Figure 4a, b). The MDA-MB-231 tumor was hypercellular, lacking a desmoplastic reaction or new bone formation. We noted that MDA-MB-231 tumor occasionally formed gland-like structures morphologically resembling human metastatic breast carcinoma. It may be that the bone microenvironment in the MDA-MB-231 tumor model has an important role in cell differentiation. This notion was also supported by various morphological tumor appearances in the soft tissue. Tumor cells in the soft tissue (e.g., muscle) were undifferentiated, resembling cells in tissue culture (Figure 4c, d).

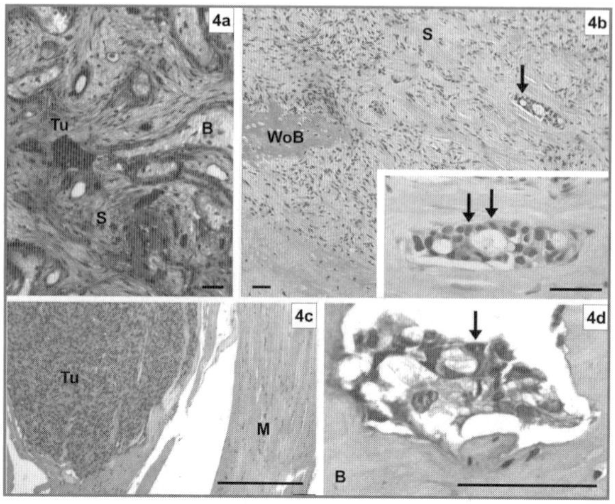

Figure 4. Comparative histological findings of bone metastasis in human specimens and experimental animal models.

(a) Undecalcified plastic-embedded human bone sample from a patient with metastatic breast carcinoma. Tumor cells and marked fibroblastic stroma surrounding the bone trabeculae (original magnification x100, Sanderson's TM Rapid Bone Stain, Van Gieson counterstain).

(b) Human specimen of metastatic breast carcinoma. Stromal new woven bone formation with gland-forming tumor nest of breast carcinoma (arrow) (original magnification x100, H&E staining). Insert- A well-preserved cribriform gland pattern of breast carcinoma (arrows) surrounded by abundant fibroblastic stroma (original magnification x400, H&E staining).

(c) MDA-MB-231 tumor. Undifferentiated tumor in the muscle compared to the tumor differentiation in bone environment (original magnification x400, H&E staining).

(d) MDA-MB-231 tumor. Gland forming metastatic tumor nest resembling human breast carcinoma (original magnification x400, H&E staining).

B-bone, BF-bone formation, LaB-lamellar bone, M-muscle, Oc-osteoclast, S-stroma, Tu-tumor, WoB-woven bone. Bar-50μm.

3. MORPHOMETRIC ALTERATIONS IN BONE METASTASIS

The numbers of quantitative morphometric studies of metastatic bone disease on human bone biopsies are still limited, especially when considering the importance of the effects of metastasis on bone loss and on bone strength. Although data from experimental animal models (19, 20, 21, 23) have provided general information about the effect of metastasis on the mechanisms of bone remodeling, the effect of tumor in humans can only be studied in human bone. Well-documented comparative reports on the morphometric changes in animal models are also relatively scarce.

3.1 Bone Histomorphometry and Node-Strut Analysis

We have previously described a bone histomorphometric method performed on bone samples obtained from patients with metastatic breast carcinoma and from animal models (12, 28). To reduce intrabone variation, we evaluated at least two sections throughout the biopsy at 100-μm intervals, at least ten microscopic fields per sections (x100 magnification).

The nomenclature and symbols used in conventional bone histomorphometry were expressed according to Parfitt et al. (29). The following parameters were measured: eroded surface (ES/BS), osteoclast surface (OcS/BS), osteoclast number per bone surface (N.Oc/BS), osteoid volume (OV/BV), osteoid surface (OS/BS), osteoblast number per bone surface (N.Ob/BS) and cancellous bone volume (BV/TV). Trabecular thickness (Tb.Th) was calculated as the BV/TV divided by half the bone surface (BS) (30, 31). Parameter related to tumor include tumor volume (TuV/TV), expressed as a fraction of total tissue volume.

Two-dimensional parameters of trabecular structure were measured by node-strut analysis according to the methods of Mellish et al. (32). The microanatomical structural parameters as indices of bone structure included: node number (N.Nd), terminus (free-end) number (N.Tm), and nodes to termini ratio (Nd/Tm). A node (Nd) was defined as a point where three or more trabeculae were joined. A terminus (Tm) was defined as the free-end of a trabecula. Node-related values are indicative of interconnectedness, and terminus-related values indicated disconnectedness of trabecular network (32, 33, 34).

3.2 Observations in Clinical Specimens

Bone resorption and bone formation are opposite ends of the spectrum of bone metabolism. We usually observed both changes simultaneously in patients with metastatic skeletal lesions. Our morphometric data suggest that bone metastases due to breast cancer amplify remodeling in predominantly quiescent bone surfaces approximately 10 fold. The dramatic increase in bone resorption was uncoupled from the subsequent bone formation phase with a net bone deficit (Table 1). This confirms that the secondary osteoblast response seen in normal bone remodeling is almost always impaired in osteolytic bone lesions (6, 35) including breast carcinoma and myeloma (8).

Table 1. Bone histomorphometric results of 33 patients with bone metastasis due to breast carcinoma.

Morphometric parameters[a]		Controls (n=20)	Metastasis (n=33)
ES/BS	(%)	1.5±0.3	26.4±4.4[b]
OcS/BS	(%)	0.4±0.1	9.4±2.6[b]
N.Oc/BS	(/mm	0.1±0.1	1.7±0.5[b]
OV/BV	(%)	0.2±0.1	1.1±0.3
OS/BS	(%)	2.0±0.5	6.9±1.6
N.Ob/BS	(/mm)	1.5±0.3	2.7±0.5
Tb Th	(μm)	121.0±11.4	85.5±4.4[b]
BV/TV	(%)	20.3±1.1	13.2±1.0[b]
WoV/BV	(%)	0	11.9±4.3
TuV/TV	(%)	0	16.8±2.5

[a]Sections of the femoral bone biopsies from patients with histologically proven breast carcinoma with bone metastases were analyzed to determine the histomorphometric parameters (mean values ± SE are shown). [b]Significantly different ($p<0.05$) from corresponding controls (Mann-Whitney U-test). See text for abbreviations of bone morphometry parameters.

Patients with bone metastases are heterogeneous with respect to the amount of bone marrow replaced by tumor tissue, bone resorption rate and the secondary osteoblastic response. Our quantitative data suggest that bone resorption and bone formation are dependent on the stage of the metastatic lesions. Osteoclastic bone resorption was quantitatively increased at earlier stages and decreased when tumor volume was higher (Figure 5). We also noticed an increase in bone formation parameters at earlier stages followed by a reduction later on. Other morphometric studies on human tissue have also suggested a decrease in both osteoclast-mediated bone resorption and new bone formation at later stages of bone destruction (6, 35, 36). Similarly, morphometric data obtained from myeloma patients have shown tumor volume-related osteoclastic bone resorption and formation (37).

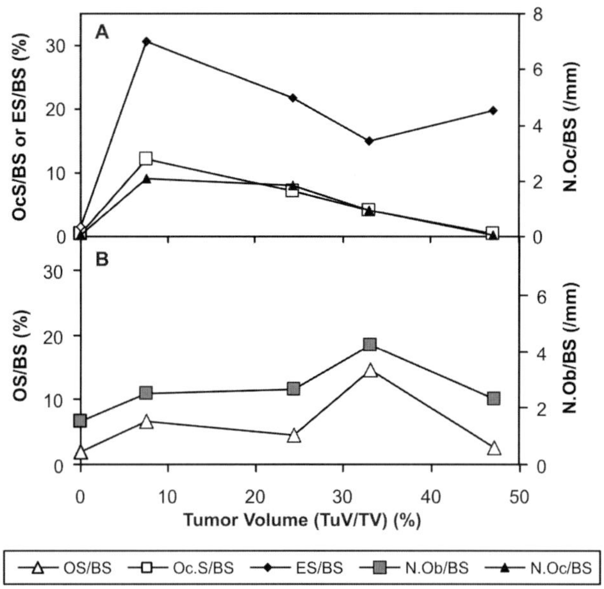

Figure 5. Biphasic osteoclastic bone resorption (A) and uncoupled bone formation (B). Tumor volume values were separated in 4 different groups with values 7.5%, 24.4%, 33%, and 47.1% respectively, to show trend of resorptive and formative parameters. Mean values and SE are shown in Table 1.

3.3 Observations in Experimental Models

Bone histomorphometry performed on metastases in animal models after intracardiac cell injection revealed significant increases in osteoclast-mediated bone resorption with a decrease in bone formation in femoral bone metastasis (Table 2). We also confirmed the morphologic observation that the MAT-LyLu spinal metastatic tumor induced a mixed, osteoblastic and osteolytic reaction, judged by the significantly increased parameters of both resorption and formation compared with controls (Table 3). Although we showed a net bone deficit, judged by the decrease in bone volume, bone histomorphometry confirmed that spinal metastasis in the MAT-LyLu model could be suitable for studying bone metastasis due to prostate carcinoma. Bone histomorphometry showed that MAT-LyLu femoral metastasis did not mimic the human situation in prostate cancer patients. However, our data obtained from spinal metastasis corresponded to previously reported morphometric evidence for bone resorption in prostate cancer patients with mixed, dominantly osteoblastic bone metastase (14).

Table 2. Bone histomorphometric results in the experimental femoral bone metastasis.

Morphometric parameters[a]	MDA-MB-231		B16/F1		Mat-LyLu	
	Controls (n=10)	Tumour (n=12)	Controls (n=10)	Tumour (n=12)	Controls (n=10)	Tumour (n=10)
ES/BS (%)	1.1±0.2	17.4±4.7[b]	0.8±0.1	6.0±1.5[b]	3.5±0.5	25.1±6.7[b]
OcS/BS (%)	0.2±0.1	6.5±1.8[b]	0.3±0.1	1.1±0.1[b]	1.6±0.26	9.7±2.1[b]
N.Oc/BS (/mm)	0.03±0.004	1.7±0.6[b]	0.1±0.01	0.7±0.1[b]	1.0±0.1	4.0±0.9[b]
OV/BV (%)	0.5±0.1	1.1±0.3	1.0±0.2	0.02±0.02[b]	0.6±0.03	0.6±0.3
OS/BS (%)	3.3±0.3	5.6±1.3	2.3±0.3	0.7±0.2[b]	1.8±0.2	1.5±0.4
N.Ob/BS (/mm)	1.9±0.2	1.8±0.5	2.0±0.4	0.7±0.2[b]	1.8±0.2	1.1±0.3
BV/TV (%)	29.5±0.3	21.2±1.1[b]	15.8±0.3	8.2±0.8[b]	21.4±0.7	18.2±2.2[b]
TbTh (μm)	104.6±7.8	78.8±10.6	62.2±7.5	32.5±2.6[b]	80.2±3.6	63.6±7.00[b]
TuV/TV (%)	0	30.3±4.1	0	77.7±18.1	0	43.8±7.5

[a]Longitudinal sections of the femora were analyzed to determine the histomorphometric parameters. [b]Significant difference ($p < 0.05$) between metastatic tumor group and corresponding control group (Mann-Whitney U test). Data represent mean ± SE of the combined values of all animals in each of the groups in three separate experiments using three different cell lines. See text for abbreviations of bone morphometry parameters.

Table 3. Bone histomorphometric results in the experimental spinal bone metastasis.

Morphometric parameters[a]	MDA-MB-231		Mat-LyLu	
	Controls (n=10)	Tumor (n=12)	Controls (n=5)	Tumor (n=5)
ES/BS (%)	0.9±0.2	14.9±2.2[b]	1.9±0.3	9.9±2.2[b]
OcS/BS (%)	0.2±0.1	6.5±1.6[b]	0.9±0.2	4.6±0.7[b]
N.Oc/BS (/mm)	0.04±0.01	2.0±0.7[b]	0.7±0.1	2.4±0.5[b]
OV/BV (%)	0.4±0.1	1.1±0.7	0.1±0.04	3.3±0.9[b]
OS/BS (%)	1.5±0.2	4.1±1.0[b]	1.0±0.3	3.3±1.0[b]
N.Ob/BS (/mm)	1.1±0.2	1.5±0.4	1.0±0.3	2.6±1.0[b]
BV/TV (%)	28.9±0.7	19.2±2.16[b]	24.0±0.8	17.5±0.9[b]
TbTh (μm)	108.9±20.0	77.1±8.0[b]	83.4±4.2	66.4±3.9
TuV/TV (%)	0	46.3±4.5	0	50.0±19.6

[a]Longitudinal sections of the spine were analyzed to determine the histomorphometric parameters. [b]Significant difference ($p<0.05$) between metastatic tumour group and corresponding control group (Mann-Whitney U test). Data represent mean ± SE of the combined values of all animals in each of the groups in three separate experiments using three different cell lines. See text for abbreviations of bone morphometry parameters.

Although MDA-MB-231 and B16/F1 tumors were both osteolytic, with significant increases in osteoclastic bone resorption parameters; there were some important differences between them. In the B16/F1 model, the tumor volume was 2.6 times greater compared to the MDA-MB-231 tumor while parameters of bone resorption were 3, 6 and 2.5 times lower for eroded surface, osteoclast bone surface and osteoclast number per bone surface, respectively. We suggested that the B16/F1 model was more suitable to study the later stages of metastatic bone disease where more than 50% of total tissue was replaced by tumor cells. We also noticed a significant reduction in bone formation parameters in this model, corresponding to later stages of human bone metastasis. We have also found that the MDA-MB-231 model was more suitable for studying the earlier stages of bone metastasis where less than 50% of the total tissue volume was replaced by tumor cells (Figure 6).

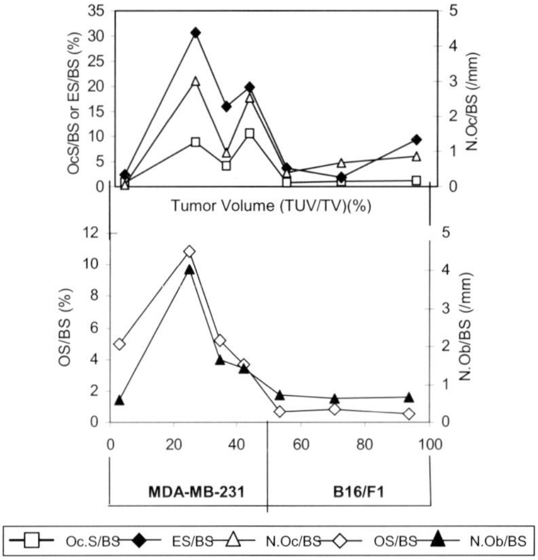

Figure 6. Comparative morphometric study on two in vivo models (MDA-MB-231 and B16/F1). Longitudinal sections of the femora were analyzed to determine histomorphometric parameters. Tumor volume values were separated in two groups (tumor volume <47% and tumor volume >47%). MDA-MB-231 tumor volume was ranging 0.4 to 42.5%. B16/F1 tumor volume was ranging from 46.3% to 95%. Mean values and SE are shown in Table 2.

Microstructural analysis based on node-strut analysis suggested different mechanisms of bone loss in the B16/F1 compared with MDA-MB-231 metastatic femoral tumor. The B16/F1 model was characterized by a significant increase in disconnectivity and irreversible bone loss with 50% reduction of bone volume. However, microstructural irreversible changes in the MDA-MB-231 bone model were manifested by a significant reduction in connectivity and 30% reduction of bone volume. Although the decrease in connectivity and increase in disconnectivity was found in the MAT-LyLu model, these differences did not reach significant values (Figure 7). Data presented here suggest that there are morphometric peculiarities of the B16/F1 metastatic bone tumor with higher tumor volume and 2.9-fold lower eroded surface compared with the MDA-MB-231 model. Although bone resorption was significantly higher than in the corresponding controls, osteoclast surface was only 18% of the eroded surface compared to 40% in the MDA-MB-231 model. However, there was a significant reduction in bone volume in both models. We suggested that osteoclastic bone resorption was not a major factor and some other cells or mechanisms were responsible for bone resorption in the B16/F1 model.

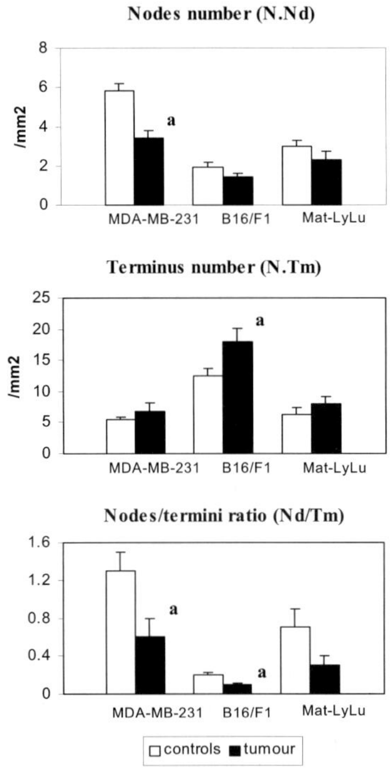

Figure 7. Results of node-strut analysis in experimental animal models. Longitudinal sections of the femora were analyzed to determine the microanatomical structural parameters described in Bone Histomorphometry and Node-Strut Analysis in the Assessment of Bone Metastasis. [a]Significant difference (p<05) between metastatic tumor and corresponding control group (Mann-Whitney U-test).

4. CONCLUSIONS

Bone metastases can be divided morphologically into three development stages: "phase of early appearance", "phase of interaction" and "phase of carcinomatosis" (8). Our quantitative data suggest that bone resorption and bone formation were dependent on the stage of metastatic bone disease in patients with metastatic breast carcinoma. Osteoclastic bone resorption was quantitatively increased at earlier stages and decreased when tumor volume was higher. We also noticed an increase in bone formation parameters at earlier stages followed by a reduction later on.

Osteoclastic bone resorption is widely accepted as quantitatively important in human metastatic breast carcinoma (7, 38, 39). Although some authors propose that tumor cells can be responsible for bone resorption, (7, 36) direct bone resorption by tumor cells is still controversial. There is in vitro evidence that breast carcinoma and prostate adenocarcinoma cells can directly degrade bone (40, 41). Tumor–mediated osteolysis by B16/F1 melanoma cells has been shown *in vivo* (27) and is described as a intertrabecular type of bone metastasis (2, 15, 16). We found that histomorphometric alterations in B16/F1 melanoma model corresponded to the later stage of metastatic bone disease where more than 50% of bone marrow was replaced by tumor cells. Data presented here indicated morphometric peculiarities of this model with higher tumor volume and lower eroded and osteoclast surface compared with the widely studied MDA-MB-231 osteolytic model. However, the B16/F1 melanoma tumor did not meet all of criteria for intertrabecular type of bone metastasis because of significant reduction in bone volume.

Bone histomorphometry techniques should serve to identify reproducible animal models of bone metastasis that mimic human bone metastasis. There is currently no animal model that fully reproduces the changes in human osteosclerotic bone metastasis. Our analysis showed site specific phenotypic differences in the murine Mat-LyLu prostate carcinoma model. Bone histomorphometry confirmed mixed type of bone metastasis in spine. However, femoral Mat-LyLu tumor was osteolytic. Data in the literature suggest that site specific differences exist showing phenotypic differences between subpopulation of osteclasts originated from intramembranous bone (calvaria) and enchondral bone (long bone) (42) leading to site specific differences between bone resorption and formation. In metastatic breast cancer patients, new bone formation is more commonly present in iliac bone compared to the femur (39).

Our morphometric data also suggested that MAT-LyLu spinal bone metastasis may be a suitable model to study metastatic prostate cancer. Although prostate metastases are bone-forming, at some point of time, osteoblastic bone formation is preceded by osteoclastic activation (25). This concept may be very important because of its potential implications for treatment with osteotropic antiresorptive agents. Similarly, comparison between fracture and non-fracture groups of metastatic patients by histomorphometry and node-strut analysis of biopsy material might also be useful for direct assessment of the effect of osteotropic drugs for prevention of bone fracture and improvement of quality of life in cancer patients.

REFERENCES

1. Coleman RE. Skeletal complications of malignancy. Cancer, 80: 1588-1594, 1997.
2. Vigorita VJ. Metastatic bone disease, pp. 472-489. In: *Orthopaedic Pathology.* V. H. Vigorita eds., Philadelphia, New York, Baltimore: Lippincott William &Wilkins, 1999.
3. Vinholes J, Coleman R, Eastell R. Effects of bone metastases on bone metabolism: implications for diagnosis, imaging and assessment of response to cancer treatment. Cancer Treat Rev, 22: 289-331, 1996.
4. Parfitt AM. Bone remodeling, normal and abnormal: a biological basis for the understanding of cancer-related bone disease and its treatment. Can J Oncol, 5 (Suppl. l): 1-10, 1995.
5. Hiraga T, Tanaka S, Ikegame M, Koizumi M, Iguchi H, Nakajima T, Ozawa H. Morphology of bone metastasis. Eur J Cancer, 34: 230-239, 1998.
6. Mundy GR. Mechanism of bone metastasis. Cancer, 80 (Suppl 8): 1546-1556, 1997.
7. Galasko CSB. Mechanism of lytic and blastic metastatic disease of bone. Clin Orthop, 169: 20-27, 1982.
8. Kulenkampff HA, Dreyer T, Kersjes W, Delling G. Histomorphometric analysis of osteoclastic bone resorption in metastatic bone disease from various primary malignomas. Virchows Arch. [Pathol Anat], 409: 817-828, 1986.
9. Kleerekoper M, Villanueva AR, Stanciu J, Sudhaker Rao D, Parfitt AM. The role of three-dimensional trabecular microstructure in the pathogenesis of vertebral compression fractures. Calcif Tissue Int, 37: 594-597, 1985.
10. Tsuchida T, Sato K, Miyakoshi N, Abe T, Kudo T, Kasukawa Y, Suzuki K. Histomorphometric evaluation of the recovering effect of human parathyroid hormone (1-34) on bone structure and turnover in streptozotocin-induced diabetic rats. Calcif Tissue Int, 66: 229-233, 2000.
11. Bross P, Reynders P, Vanderschot P. Surgical treatment of the metastatic fracture of the femur improves quality of life. Acta Orthop Belg, 59 (Suppl 1): 52-56, 1993.
12. Vukmirovic-Popovic S, Colterjohn N, Lhotak S, Duivenvoorden WC, Orr FW, Singh G. Morphological, histomorphometric, and microstructural alterations in human bone metastasis from breast carcinoma. Bone, 31: 529-535, 2002.
13. Coindre JM, Mage P, Bui BN, Goussot JF, De Mascarel A, Trojani M. Prostatic osteocondensing metastases and osteomalacia. Value of histomorphometric study. Preliminary results. Presse Med, 14: 1823-1827, 1985.

14. Hiraga T, Mundy GR, Yoneda T. Bone metastases-morphology, pp. 65-74. In: *Cancer and the Skeleton.* R. D. Rubens and G. R. Mundy eds, London: Martin Dunitz Ltd, 2000.
15. Yamaguchi T, Tamai K, Yamato M, Honma K, Ueda Y, Saotome K. Intertrabecular pattern of tumours metastatic to bone. Cancer, 78: 1388-1394, 1996.
16. Fornasier VL, Horne JG. Metastases to the vertebral column. Cancer, 36: 590-594, 1975.
17. McCarthy EF, Frassica FJ. Metastatic carcinoma in bone, pp. 175-183. In: *Pathology of bone and joint disorders with Clinical and Radiographic Correlation.* McCarthy EF, Frassica FJ, eds, Philadelhia, PA: W. B. Saunders, 1998.
18. Clarke NW, McClure J, George NJR. Morphometric evidence for bone resorption and replacement in prostate cancer. Br J Urol, 68: 74-80, 1991.
19. Arguello FB, Baggs RB, Frantz CN. A murine model of experimental metastasis to bone and bone marrow. Cancer Res, 48: 6876-6881, 1988.
20. Yoneda T. Arterial microvascularization and breast cancer colonization in bone. Histol Histopathol, 12: 1145-1149, 1997.
21. Yoneda T, Michigami T, Yi B, Williams PJ, Niewolna M, Hiraga T. Action of bisphosphonate on bone metastasis in animal models of breast carcinoma. Cancer, 88: 2979-2988, 2000.
22. Sasaki A, Boyce BF, Story B, Wright KR, Chapman M, Boyce R, Mundy GR, Yoneda T. Bisphosphonate risedronate reduces metastatic human breast cancer burden in bone in nude mice. Cancer Res, 55: 3551-3557, 1995.
23. Sasaki A, Kitamura K, Alcalde RE, Tanaka T, Suzuki A, Etoh Y, Matsumura T. Effect of a newly developed bisphosphonate, YH529, on osteolytic bone metastases in nude mice. Int J Cancer, 77: 279-285, 1998.
24. Nemeth JA, Harb JF, Barroso U Jr, He Z, Grignon DJ, Cher ML. Severe combined immunodeficient-hu model of human prostate cancer metastasis to human bone. Cancer Res, 59: 1987-1993, 1999.
25. Nemeth JE, Yousif R, Herzog M, Che M, Upadhyay J, Shekarriz B, Bhagat S, Mullins C, Fridman R, Cher ML. Matrix metalloproteinase activity, bone matrix turnover, and tumour cell proliferation in prostate cancer bone metastasis. J Natl Cancer Inst, 94: 17-25, 2002.
26. Rabbani SA, Harakidas P, Davidson DJ, Henkin J, Mazar AP. Prevention of prostate-cancer metastasis in vivo by novel synthetic inhibitor of urokinase-type plasminogene activator (uPA). Int J Cancer, 63: 840-845, 1995.
27. Sanchez-Sweatman OH, Lee J, Orr FW, Singh G. Direct osteolysis induced by metastatic murine melanoma cells: of matrix metalloproteinases. Eur J Cancer, 33: 918-925, 1997.
28. Duivenvoorden WC, Vukmirovic Popovic S, Lhotak S, Seidlitz E, Hirte H W, Tozer RG, Singh G. Doxycycline decreases tumour burden in a bone metastasis model of human breast cancer. Cancer Res, 62: 1588-1591, 2002.
29. Parfitt AM, Drezner MK, Glorieux FH, Kanis JA, Malluche H, Meunier PJ, Ott SM, Recker RR. Bone histomorphometry: Standardization of nomenclature, symbols, and units. Report of the ASBMR Histomorphometry Nomenclature Committee. J. Bone Min Res, 2: 595-610, 1987.
30. Parfitt AM. Stereological basis of bone histomorphometry: Theory of quantitative microscopy and reconstruction of the third dimension, pp. 61-64. In: *Bone*

histomorphometry: techniques and interpretation. R. R. Recker eds., Florida: Boca Raton, CRC Press, 1982.

31. Parfitt AM, Mathews CH, Villanueva AR, Kleerekope, M, Frame BR. Relationships between surface, volume, and thickness of iliac trabecular bone in aging and in osteoporosis. Implications for the microanatomic and cellular mechanisms of bone loss. J Clin Invest, 72: 1396-1409, 1983.
32. Melish RWE, Ferguson-Pell, MW, Cochran GV, Lindsay R, Dempster DW. A new manual method for assessing two-dimensional cancellous bone structure: comparison between iliac crest and lumbar vertebra. J Bone Miner Res, 6: 689-696, 1991.
33. Carbonare LD, Arlot, ME, Chavassieux JP, Roux JP, Portero NR, Meunier PJ. Comparison of trabecular bone microarchitecture and remodeling in glucocorticoid-induced and postmenopausal osteoporosis. J Bone Miner Res, 16:97-103, 2001.
34. Zhang L, Takahashi HE, Inoue J, Tanizawa T, Endo N, Yamamoto N, Hori M. Effect of intermittent administration of low dose human PTH (1-34) on cancellous and cortical bone of lumbar vertebral bodies in adult beagles. Bone, 21: 501-506, 1997.
35. Mundy GR, Guise TA. Pathophysiology of bone metastasis, pp. 43-64. In: *Cancer and the Skeleton.* Rubens RD, Mundy GR, eds, London: Martin Dunitz, 2000.
36. Galasko CSB. Mechanism of bone destruction in the development of skeletal metastases. Nature, 263: 507-508, 1976.
37. Taube T, Beneton MNC, McCloskey EV, Rogers S, Greaves M, Kanis JA. Abnormal bone remodeling in patients with myelomatosis and normal biochemical indices of bone resorption. Eur J Haematol, 49: 192-198, 1992.
38. Taube T, Elomaa I, Blomqvist C, Beneton MNC, Kanis JA. Comparative effects of clodronate and calcitonin on bone in metastatic breast cancer: A histomorphometric study. Eur J Cancer, 29A/12: 1677-1681, 1993.
39. Taube T, Elomaa I, Blomqvist C, Beneton MNC, Kanis JA. Histomorphometric evidence for osteoclast-mediated bone resorption in metastatic breast cancer. Bone, 15: 161-166, 1994.
40. Eilon G, Mundy GR. Direct resorption of bone by human breast cancer cells in vitro. Nature, 276: 726-729, 1978.
41. Sanchez-Swetman OH, Orr FW, Singh G. Human metastatic prostate PC3 cell lines degrade bone using matrix metalloproteinases. Invasion Metastasis, 18: 297-305, 1998-1999.
42. Everts V, Korper W, Jansen DC, Steinfort J, Lammerse I, Heera S, Docherty AJ, Beertsen W. Functional heterogeneity of osteoclasts: matrix metalloproteinases participate in osteoclastic resorption of calvarial bone but not in resorption of long bone. FASEB J, 13: 1219-1230, 1999.

Chapter 4

CLINICAL MODALITIES FOR THE DIAGNOSIS, CHARACTERIZATION AND DETECTION OF BONE METASTASES

Michael H. Weber[1,4], Jonathan C. Sharp[4], Thomas H. Hassard[2], Martin Reed[5], James A. Thliveris[3], F. William Orr[1]
[1]The Department of Pathology, University of Manitoba, Winnipeg, Manitoba, Canada; [2]Department of Community Health Science, University of Manitoba, Winnipeg, Manitoba, Canada; [3]Department of Human Anatomy and Cell Science; [4]Institute for Biodiagnostics, National Research Council of Canada, Winnipeg, Manitoba, Canada; [5]The Department of Radiology, Health Sciences Centre, Winnipeg, Manitoba, Canada

1. INTRODUCTION

1.1 Clinical Significance

Breast cancer is a leading cause of death in women, occurring in one of eight during their lifetime. A comparable cancer in men, prostate cancer, claims the lives of just under 30,000 men in the United States each year with a prevalence of one in six (1). These tumors, along with carcinomas of the lung, thyroid, and kidney have a high propensity to metastasize to bone, which constitutes one of their most serious complications, creates a great challenge for treatment, and often carries a poor prognosis. Metastases are the most frequent bone tumors and cause significant morbidity due to pain, osteolysis, pathological fractures, hypercalcemia, and anemia (2). Established bone metastases are resistant to treatment and current therapeutic approaches such as endocrine therapy, radiation therapy, and chemotherapy are often ineffective (3). This chapter has been written on the premise that a

G. Singh and W. Orr (eds.), Bone Metastasis and Molecular Mechanisms, 49-69.

better understanding of the pathophysiology of bone metastasis may provide insight into the design of diagnostic techniques that would help to identify bone metastasis formation at its earliest stages. This may provide an opportunity for early treatment and alleviate the necessity to treat them at a late stage.

1.2 Pathophysiology

The majority of bone metastases arise from a hematogenous route. The venous system, as opposed to the arterial system is especially important in Batson's paravertebral plexus. The axial skeleton and proximal long bones are two sites with high propensity for metastatic involvement because of Batson's plexus communications and the greater vascularity of red marrow as opposed to yellow marrow found in these anatomic locations (4, 5).

There is strong evidence that the formation of bone metastases is the result of a synergistic relationship between cancer cells and the unique environment within the osseous microcompartment (Figure 1). Osteolysis is a dominant feature of most established metastases and is widely recognised to be the consequence of osteoclastic bone resorption. Many cancer cells secrete parathyroid hormone-related protein which will promote the osteoblasts to initiate osteoclastogenesis utilizing the receptor activator of NF-κB (RANK) and its ligand (RANKL) (6, 7). The multinucleated osteoclasts, derivatives of their monocytic precursors, resorb bone, releasing growth factors and cytokines, including transforming growth factor-β (TGF-β), which in turn can stimulate proliferation of metastatic cells via Smad and MAP kinase pathways, reinforcing this pathological cycle (8). There is evidence that some metastatic cells can induce bone resorption directly by secreting matrix metalloproteinases (9).

Cells from prostate cancer can induce osteosclerosis. Mediators of osteoblastic reactions include endothelin-1, TGF-β, fibroblast growth factor and endothelial growth factor (EGF) which can stimulate osteoblasts to initiate bone formation [reviewed by Guise et al., 2003 (10)]. A second pathway involves secretion of proteinases, prostate specific antigen and urokinase plasminogen activator, which can activate latent TGF-β and inactivate parathyroid hormone-related protein (11, 12).

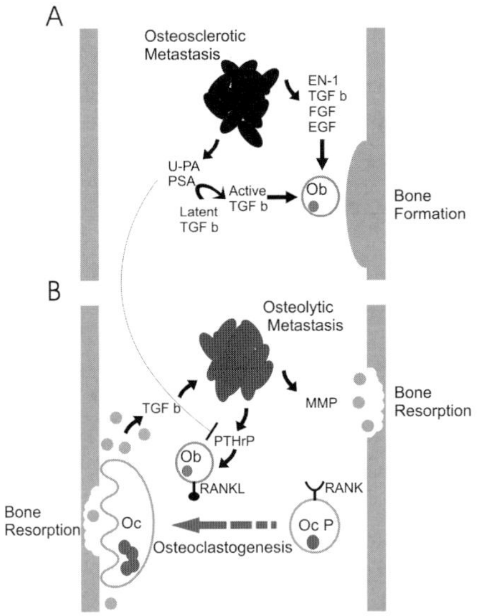

Figure 1. Current concepts relating to the pathophysiology of bone metastases. A diagrammatic representation of bone metastasis induced (A) osteosclerosis and (B) osteolysis. Parathyroid hormone-related protein (PTHrP), Receptor activator of NF-κB (RANK), Receptor activator of NF-κB ligand (RANKL), Matrix metalloproteinases (MMP), Endothelin-1 (EN-1), Transforming growth factor-β (TGFβ), Fibroblast growth factor (FGF), Endothelial growth factor (EGF), Prostate specific antigen (PSA), Urokinase plasminogen activator (U-PA), Osteoblasts (Ob), Osteoclasts (Oc), and Osteoclast precursor (OcP).

1.3 Detection

Insightful interpretation of results from various detection techniques is dependent on understanding the pathophysiology of bone metastasis development. Metastatic bone disease ranges from colonization of the marrow by micrometastatic cells to clinically significant bone metastases and resulting changes to bone microanatomy. Single micrometastatic epithelial cells in a mesenchymal bone marrow cavity are distinguishable using immunocytochemistry, flow cytometry and molecular techniques. Biochemical markers may be used to directly detect and monitor changes in normal bone metabolism due to the effects of metastases on the normal balance between bone formation and resorption. Diagnostic imaging techniques such as plain radiography, bone scintigraphy and magnetic resonance imaging directly identify late stage clinically significant metastases and the resulting change in the bone architecture.

The detection of bone metastases is intimately dependent on the pathophysiology of the primary tumor. The three modalities investigated in this chapter for the detection, quantification, and further understanding of the development of bone metastases and response to therapy include the use of tumor specific molecular markers, identification of serum levels of biochemical markers, and radiological identification.

2. MOLECULAR MARKERS

Bone marrow and blood are both relatively accessible and have been frequently surveyed for the presence of disseminated tumor cells in patients with solid tumors. Blood represents the vehicle for the hematogenous spread of disseminated tumor cells to bone (13). Bone marrow acts as a filter and is a preferential environment for the eventual growth of disseminated tumor cells (14). Small aggregates of tumor cells have been observed using standard cytologic and histologic methods (15) and some workers have identified single disseminated tumor cells (16). The cellular aggregates may have greater malignant potential than single disseminated tumor cells (17-19, 20). Despite the cross reactivity of membrane antigens with hematopoietic cells, immunocytochemical tests using monoclonal antibodies to epithelial-specific antigens have been created to identify disseminated tumor cells in the bone and peripheral blood (21-23). The non-epithelial nature of blood and bone marrow make it ideal for the differentiation of epithelial derived tumor cells using epithelial-specific proteins (23, 24), RNA expression (25-27), and tumor-specific DNA abnormalities (28, 29). For a review, see Zippelius and Pantel (30).

The goal of most detection techniques is good sensitivity and specificity. To improve specificity the marker must not be present in the background hematopoietic cells. However using both tumor specific antibodies (31) and RT-PCR (32, 33) false positives have been reported. Quality control is key to decreasing crossover contamination and amplification of non-specific and pseudogenes. To improve sensitivity, a number of markers may need to be screened to avoid false negatives (34-36).

The current convention is to use molecular markers to identify disseminated tumor cells (37, 24) as well as to characterize these cells for an improved knowledge of the pathophysiology of bone metastases (38). These approaches have led to the identification of critical proteins and/or genes involved in bone metastasis development. Disseminated tumor cells, collected from cancer patients, have a metastatic phenotype (39), elevated proliferation potential (40) and can generate metastases in mice (41). The ability of disseminated tumor cells to act as seeds for clinically significant metastases is substantiated by both the long dormancy of residual cancer cells and by the transmission of cancer after organ transplant (42, 43).

However, the presence of disseminated tumor cells in blood or marrow does not always predict the eventual formation of clinically significant bone metastases (44). It has been demonstrated with follow-up sampling that there is a clearance of disseminated tumor cells after surgery (45). Moreover, it is likely that the majority of disseminated single metastatic tumor cells in bone do not proliferate (46). Only a few large long-term follow-up studies have been carried out (44, 47). As a prognostic indicator, the presence of disseminated tumor cells is at best comparable to established staging techniques (48). In addition, the number of patients with disseminated tumor cells varies from study to study (49, 50). A standard detection technique is critical for the accurate comparison of studies (51). For example the prognostic significance of disseminated tumor cells in blood may (52) or may not (24) be comparable to that of bone marrow. This may in part be due to the difference in definition of prognosis from the number of patients with disseminated tumor cells who will develop clinically significant metastases to the five-year survival rates. Sampling time with reference to when the surgical procedure is conducted is crucial, affecting both the number and characteristics of the disseminated tumor cells (45, 53). To reduce sampling error more than one sample is required to accurately test for the presence and characteristics of scarce and inhomogeneously localized disseminated tumor cells (54).

3. BIOCHEMICAL MARKERS

Biochemical markers expressed by neoplastic cells, such as carcinoembryonic antigen (CEA), tissue polypeptide antigen (TPA), and the carbohydrate antigen (CA 125), have been used to identify patients with a number of primary tumors that have a propensity to metastasize to bone including breast, ovary, lung, and prostate cancer. Some of these markers have been used to monitor the response of bone metastases to therapy (55-57). Regretfully, the ability of CEA, TPA and CA 125 to diagnoses bone metastases has been inconsistent when compared with markers for bone turnover (58, 59). Prostate specific antigen (PSA) is a widely used biochemical marker, not only for diagnosis and follow-up of prostate cancer, but also for evidence of prostatic bone metastases (60, 61). A level of PSA more than 100 μg/l indicates a high probability of bone metastases, however the sensitivity of this cutoff is inconsistent, from 42.9% to 83.3% (62, 63, 64).

adequate for true osteolytic lesions and therefore useful to assess fracture risk, however the method is less useful to identify mixed lytic-blastic metastases (82).

4.2 Computed Tomography (CT)

Unlike radiography, computed tomography (CT) is not limited by low contrast resolution and by the obscuring effect of superimposed bone and soft tissue. CT offers a higher sensitivity (83) and earlier detection of lytic changes in trabecular bone than radiography (84). On CT, bone metastases have an increased attenuation value compared to the fat containing marrow, and because of this, CT is an effective modality for the differentiation between benign and malignant lesions observed on bone scintigraphy (85). Although CT has been reported to be an effective means of evaluating bone metastases in the skeleton because of its sensitivity compared to plain film x-ray (86, 87), CT is a very awkward method for screening of the entire skeleton.

4.3 Bone Scintigraphy

Bone scintigraphy is twice as sensitive as radiography (88) and enables the scanning of the entire skeleton in a short period of time. Bone scintigraphy is used as a screening technique for the detection of bone metastases primarily due to its high sensitivity and acceptable specificity (59). However, $^{99}Tc^{m}$-phosphorous compounds do not specifically associate with tumor cells or offer information on the osteolytic process. Instead these complexes are incorporated into hydroxyapatite crystals as a result of new bone formation, a nonspecific response of normal bone to a pathological process. A metastatic lesion, a fracture, infection, inflammation, or degenerative change, typically appears as areas of increased uptake compared to the normal surrounding bone.

Rigorous evaluation of the disease process is limited and only progression can be identified reliably with bone scintigraphy. However, as with plain radiography, a lag time of six to eight months is also required before sufficiently gross changes will become evident with scintigraphic findings (89, 90). The use of bone scans for assessment of the response to therapy is unreliable, primarily due to the flare phenomenon, which is a consequence of an initial increase in bone formation in patients responding to systemic therapy (91). Bone scintigraphy cannot differentiate between tumor progression and the flare phenomenon (92) or provide information on the extent of individual lesions.

4.4 Magnetic Resonance Imaging (MRI)

Magnetic resonance imaging (MRI) provides a digitized image with contrast based upon the hydrogen nuclei concentration (proton density) and proton interaction with neighboring molecules (T1 and T2 relaxation)[1]. Hydrogen protons are most plentiful in water and fat. Water and fat have opposing signal intensities and as such on T1-weighted images, fat gives a high signal and water a low signal, while on T2-weighted images, water offers a high signal and fat a low signal. Pathology, such as bone metastases, changes the relative water and fat concentration, thereby producing contrast (93, 94).

MRI is the most sensitive and only imaging modality to allow direct visualization of the marrow (95). MRI can discriminate between bone metastases and non-neoplastic lesions, such as osteoporotic compression fractures, degenerative lesions (96-98), and inflammatory responses. MRI can detect bone metastases that are not apparent on radioisotope bone scans because it can detect an intramedullary lesion before destruction of the cortex, and before an osteoblastic reaction is detected on bone scan (99, 100). In particular, MRI is superior to planar scintigraphy in its ability to detect spinal metastases due to the difficulty of planar scintigraphy to recognize subtle radionuclide abnormalities (101, 102). More recently, single photon emission computed tomography (SPECT) has been shown to be more beneficial in the detection of single vertebral metastases than planar bone scans (103), and argued by some authors to be comparable to MRI (104).

The sensitivity of MRI is high, so to improve specificity, an appropriate choice of an acquisition pulse sequence is required. Spin-echo offers good signal-to-noise ratio and contrast of bone and metastatic lesions. The need for rapid and effective sequences to survey the entire skeleton for signs of metastases has resulted in fast spin-echo and inversion recovery image sequences development (105). Our published studies have demonstrated that high resolution MRI is an effective means for the quantitative evaluation of the normal variation in bone microanatomy as compared to a histological "gold standard", and a superior means of quantification in comparison to micro x-ray (Figure 2) (106).

[1] T1 and T2 relaxation are defined as the time required for the excited protons to return to equilibrium and diphase, respectively (133).

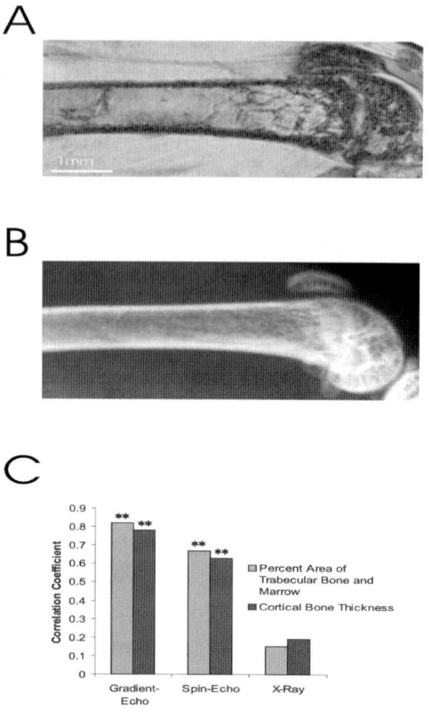

Figure 2. Representative images of a distal femur from a C57bl/6 mouse. (A) Longitudinal gradient-echo image from an 11.7T MR microscopy scanner with in-plane resolution of 35μm. Note the detail MRI provides of the marrow micro-architecture. (B) High-resolution x-ray of a distal femur from a C57bl/6 mouse. (C) Details of a comparison between cortical bone thickness, percent marrow and trabecular bone data from the histological gold standard and data from an 11.7T MR microscopy scanner and x-ray. * and **indicate significance between quantified MRI and histological data at $p \leq 0.01$ and $p \leq 0.001$, respectively, by a Multiple Regression test.

In the human adult, the majority of the marrow is yellow or fat-containing. On T1-weighted spin-echo MR images, fat has high signal intensity, and water and bone metastases low signal intensity (except for some rare lipoblastic metastases). Bone metastases can often be differentiated from low intensity focal areas of red hematopoeitic marrow on T1-weighted MR images since red marrow has a lower signal intensity than fat but a higher signal intensity than normal muscles, is normally uniformly demarcated, and can have centrally located fat (107).

The difference in resonance frequency between water and fat protons can be useful for the detection of metastases. Bone metastases appear using a fat-suppressed T1-weighted image as mixed to high intensity (108). Short tau inversion recovery (STIR) and out-of-phase acquisitions improve the contrast between metastases and normal bone marrow (109).

Bone metastases are significantly brighter than background marrow with T2-weighted spin-echo images due to the higher water content in these lesions. In addition, bone metastases can have a diagnostic rim of bright T2 signal, forming the circumference of the metastases (107). Diffusion weighted spin-echo imaging is reported to be no better than non-contrast enhanced T1 weighted imaging, but is advantageous over T2 weighted imaging (110).

Gradient-echo sequences show metastases as more homogeneous and higher in signal intensity than normal marrow, and also enable direct visualization of the resultant changes in bone. Because of a lack of mobile protons, trabecular bone offers no detectable signal and generates local field heterogeneity. The heterogeneous magnetic field has little effect on spin-echo sequences because of the correcting 180° pulse. The gradient-echo sequence cannot compensate for field heterogeneity thus leading to signal cancellation and loss (111-114). As the echo time (TE) is lengthened, signal can decrease markedly in regions of bone with increased trabecular bone. This is of clinical relevance when trabecular lysis occurs as a result of metastatic disease since the signal will become higher than the rest of the bone.

In an attempt to improve on this, a number of contrast agents have been used. There is no observable (<10%) change in normal marrow with the injection of gadolinium chelates on T1-weighted images (115, 116). Bone metastases typically have a strong signal increase with the injection of gadolinium chelates, however this is not pathognomonic because a similar change is seen in infectious or inflammatory reactions. Supermagnetic iron oxide particles are taken up by macrophages and markedly decrease the T2 in normal marrow (117). However, in neoplastic bone marrow there is only a minor or no signal decline (118).

5. CONCLUSION

Metastatic bone tumors are the most common type of malignant bone lesion, and bone is the third most frequent metastatic site after the lung and liver (119). The molecular mechanisms responsible for the spread and survival of metastatic tumor cells are unclear. Ideally, these single micrometastatic cells would represent preferable targets for treatment, compared to established late stage bone metastases where there is a much larger tumor cell population and extensive alteration in the bone architecture. Hypothetically, therapeutic intervention at this early stage would benefit significant numbers of macrophages and endothelial cells. Advantages and disadvantages are attached to this approach, namely the creation of a composite *in vitro* cellular environment to some extent reminiscent of the *in vivo* situation, and the inability to model the direct interaction of the cancer cell with the stromal cell proper.

Instrumental in the ability to isolate bone marrow stromal cells directly from marrow by FACS has been the development and characterization of the mouse monoclonal antibody, Stro-1 (17, 18). The population of Stro-1 positive cells isolated from single cell suspensions of bone marrow effectively isolates virtually all of the CFU-F that can be enumerated by using the classic "colony forming efficiency" assay developed by Friedenstein (19). This assay relies on the ability of a stromal cell to become quickly adherent (unlike most hematopoietic cells, murine macrophages being the exception), and to proliferate to form a colony. However, approximately 1% of marrow cells are Stro-1 positive, a proportion far higher than the frequency of CFU-F calculated from adherent assays (~10-20 cells per 10^5 marrow mononuclear cells). Closer examination reveals that the Stro-1 population can be further subdivided based on intensity. The majority of the cells are Stro-1^{dull} and are primarily erythroblasts, whereas Stro-1^{bright} cells include all of the adherent clonogenic cells, yet not all Stro-1^{bright} cells are clonogenic (20). Stro-1^{bright} populations co-express a variety of integrins, including $\alpha_1\beta_1$, $\alpha_2\beta_1$, $\alpha_5\beta_1$, $\alpha_6\beta_1$, $\alpha_v\beta_3$ and $\alpha_v\beta_5$, while only a proportion of stromal precursors expressed the integrin $\alpha_4\beta_1$, and no measurable levels of the integrin $\alpha_3\beta_1$ were detected (21).

It was subsequently found that the Stro-1^{bright} population could be further purified by dual-color cell sorting using Stro-1 and VACM-1 (CD106) (20), and others have used similar approaches using other surface markers. The Stro1^{bright}/VCAM-1 population was negative for the hematopoietic marker, CD34. Of note, 90% of these cells expressed type I collagen, whereas 70% expressed alpha-smooth muscle actin. The dual sorted population was uniformly negative for the osteogenic transcription factors (CBFA1 and Osterix) markers of mature osteoblastic cells (osteopontin and osteocalcin), and chrondrocytes (type II collagen and aggrecan), but interestingly, routinely expressed type X collagen, a hypertrophic chondrocyte marker. In evaluation of markers of adipogenic commitment and differentiation, only LDL was expressed.

Explantation of bone marrow stromal cells *in vitro*, even those "purified" by FACS, reveals the inherent heterogeneity of the population. When seeded at high density and analyzed en mass, they are uniformly negative for hematopoietic markers. Some cells within the population display some, characteristics of endothelial cells such as CD146 (MUC-18, Mel-CAM), and endoglin, but notably are negative for Factor VIII (22). Virtually all express type I collagen, but are variably positive for other connective tissue and osteogenic markers such as osteonectin, alkaline phosphatase, osteopontin, bone sialoprotein and osteocalcin. The same variability is noted in expression of adipogenic markers such as CEBP-alpha, PPAR-gamma2, and leptin. Interestingly, and in keeping with their potential origin as perivascular cells, some express smooth muscle markers such as alpha-smooth muscle actin and the pericyte marker, 3G5 (9,23). When plated at low density, the heterogeneity is even more pronounced in the colonies that are formed by individual CFU-Fs. Cells with different morphologies such as a large and flat cells, spindle-shaped fibroblastic cells, and a range of morphologies in between these two extremes develop colonies that grow at different rates and with different habits. In some cases, the cells are highly migratory and remain in monolayer, while others form multi-layers and display evidence of osteoblastic differentiation (24). Yet, extensive analysis of morphology, histochemical markers, patterns of gene expression and in vivo transplantation of such clonally derived strains has failed to determine the "fingerprint" by which a colony can be determined to be multi-potential *a priori* (25).

6. STROMAL CELL-CANCER CELL INTERACTIONS

There are several possible mechanisms by which bone marrow stroma mediates cancer metastasis to bone involving chemotaxis, cell-matrix, cell-cell and cell-factor interactions. It has been proposed that chemoattractant factors emanate from the marrow as a result of bone turnover, such as type I collagen degradation fragments, or products of stromal cells themselves Stromal derived factor-1, and growth factors such as TGF-beta, IGF-1 and 2, and osteonectin, attract cancer cells in the blood stream to adhere to the microvasculature and extravasate (26). Once in the extravascular spaces, cancer cells encounter a distinctly unusual extraceullar matrix that is composed of thin reticular fibers of types I, III and V collagens, presumably oriented by chondroitin and heparin sulfate proteoglycans, fibronectin and thrombospondin, and held within a gel-like substance composed primarily of hyaluronic acid. Although there are a number of studies describing the interaction of cancer cells with various different matrix components *in vitro*, the interactions of cancer cells with matrix as it exists *in situ* remain to be characterized.

Direct cell-cell contact undoubtedly mediates a number of events in the establishment of a metastasis, although not well defined to date. It is possible that molecules that govern stromal cell-hematopoietic cell interactions [integrins, selectins, the immunoglobulin superfamily, and mucin-like molecules, reviewed in (27)] may also be operative in stromal-cancer cell interactions. Based on the expression of CD44, a hyaluronic acid receptor, by both hematopoietic progenitor cells and myeloma cells, it had been assumed that tumor cells (in particular, with variant forms of CD44) interact with hyaluronic acid in the extravascular spaces. More recent findings suggest that the receptor binds directly to an as yet unidentified ligand on stromal cells (28), which in turn stimulates the production of IL-6 by stromal cells (29).

Finally, it is clear that cell-factor interactions have a profound effect on progression of metastatic bone disease. Metastatic cells in the marrow microenvironment are bathed in a rich milieu of growth factors and cytokines including (but not limited to) bFGF, IGFs, PDGF, EFG, TGF-beta and BMPs that are capable of stimulating cancer cell growth, as in prostate cancer. (30, 31). Furthermore, these stromal-derived factors induce cancer cell expression of factors such as PTHrP, IL-1, IL-6, IL-11 and TNF-alpha and beta (32), which are known to stimulate the formation and activity of osteoclasts. PTHrP, in particular, has been implicated in stromal cell expression of RANKL, an essential component for initiation of osteoclast formation (33). Furthermore, many of these cytokines induce a variety of proteinases in stromal cells and cancer cells alike, although a full description of the patterns of induction is not available. Thus, the interplay between stromal cells and cancer cells results in the establishment of an osteolytic process, characteristic of end stages of most types of metastatic bone disease (34).

7. STROMAL CELLS AND THE MODELING OF BONE METASTASIS

Either multi-colony-derived strains or some single colony-derived (clonal) strains of *ex-vivo* expanded marrow stromal cells are able to generate, when transplanted in the subcutaneous tissue of immunocompromised mice, a host of connective tissues of donor origin, including bone, adipose tissue, fibrous tissue, a reticular-fibroblastic stroma capable of supporting hematopoiesis, and also, under specific experimental conditions, cartilage. These tissues are organized in an orderly structure, which overall, faithfully recapitulates the structure of any anatomical site with a trabecular bone/bone marrow structure. Furthermore, the marrow spaces formed among the bony trabeculae become colonized by a complete hematopoietic tissue, in which all major lineages undergo a normal differentiation/maturation sequence. Experiments using markers of species origin of the different tissues (e.g., *in situ* hybridization experiments employing probes specific for human specific Alu sequences) have demonstrated that while the bony structures and the associated stromal tissues are of donor origin, the hematopoietic cells colonizing the ectopic miniature of a skeletal site (also called the "ectopic ossicle") are of host origin (15,19). Thus, the transplanted cells generate not only bone, but also a hematopoietic microenvironment, which then becomes seeded by blood-borne murine hematopoietic stem cells, which in turn generate a hematopoietic tissue (35). In these systems, thus, the classical "seed-and-soil" paradigm underlying the normal ontogeny of the bone/bone marrow organ [and also, as recognized by Stephen Paget as early as 1889, for the ontogeny of bone metastasis, (1)] is reproduced, and the ultimate outcome of the procedure essentially represents a mirror image of the chimeric bone marrow generated by transplantation of hematopoietic progenitors also in humans (where the hematopoietic cells are of donor origin, and the stroma is of host origin) – indeed, a true "reverse" bone marrow transplantation (36).

Multi-potent progenitors capable of self-renewal and of generation of both bone tissue and a hematopoietic microenvironment represent bona fide skeletal stem cells, whereas cells capable of more restricted differentiation capacity, limited to the ability of generating bone tissue, but not bone marrow stroma, upon transplantation, are regarded as committed osteogenic progenitors (4). Both types of progenitors may participate in the osteogenic response to cancer metastasis. However, short-lived, default osteogenesis occurring in virtually all metastasis, and sustained osteosclerosis restricted to specific types of bone metastasis may involve the recruitment and activation of distinct osteogenic progenitors in the bone marrow. This, in turn, may be rooted into the specific biological activity of cancer cells.

In vivo transplantation assay forms the basic experimental approach to the investigation of the differentiation and organogenic potential of skeletal stem cells under normal conditions, and of their use on a larger scale for tissue engineering and cell therapy of skeletal tissues (37). We have shown that these systems can also be bent to the investigation of genetic diseases of the skeleton, by transplanting strains of human skeletal progenitor cells derived from the bone marrow of patients carrying specific genetic anomalies. In this type of application, mutated human skeletal progenitor cells generate miniature replicas of specific human skeletal diseases of known genotype (38,39), or of unknown genotype (40). Likewise, transplanted skeletal stem cells effectively demonstrate the cell-autonomous skeletal effects of targeted mutations of murine genes (41). Thus, these systems have a specific value in investigating human diseases and in generating advanced models thereof.

This system can provide a valuable model for investigating mechanisms of the homing of cancer cells to the human bone/bone marrow environment, an essential step in the development of bone metastasis. The very fact that the ectopic skeletal tissues become colonized by murine hematopoietic cells proves that blood-borne (hematopoietic) cells capable of recognizing the specific bone microenvironment can be home to the ectopic environment with similar efficiency as to the orthotopic bone. Thus, one can envision that cancer cells inoculated intravenously in animals bearing an ectopic ossicle would seek the ectopic human bone marrow microenvironment, seed it, and develop into an ectopic mini-metastasis in human bone. The resulting model would have two significant fallouts. The availability of human bone and marrow as homing sites would permit modeling of metastasis of tumor types that do not efficiently seed mouse bone, such as prostate cancer. Thus, a model of prostate cancer metastasis for conventional studies including those aiming at bone changes (e.g., induction of osteoclastic bone resorption, or stimulation of excess bone formation) or drug testing would become available. The other and more significant one derives from the fact that the bone environment itself, in the envisioned system, is built *de novo*, *in vivo*, with cells previously isolated and expanded in culture. This means that the system allows for the manipulation of both partners of the cancer cell/stromal cell interaction, thus setting the stage for an *in vivo* experimental approach to the molecular mechanisms of their interaction.

ACKNOWLEDGEMENTS

PB gratefully acknowledges the support of the Associazione Italiana per la Ricerca sul Cancro (AIRC)

REFERENCES

1. Paget S. The distribution of secondary growths in cancer of the breast. Lancet 1, 571-573, 1889.
2. Bianco P, Riminucci M. The bone marrow stroma in vivo: ontogeny, structure, cellular composition and changes in disease, pp. 10-25. In: *Marrow Stromal Cell Cultures.* Beresford JN, Owen M, eds., Cambridge, U.K., Cambridge University Press, 1998.
3. Tavassoli M, Yoffey JM., eds. Bone Marrow: Structure and Function. New York, NY, Alan R. Liss, Inc., 1983.

4. Bianco P, Robey PG. Skeletal stem cells. In: *Handbook of Adult and Fetal Stem Cells.* R. Lanza, ed, San Diego, CA, Elsevier, in press.
5. Bianco P, Boyde A. Confocal images of marrow stromal (Westen-Bainton) cells. Histochemistry, 100: 93-99, 1993.
6. Bianco P, Bradbeer JN, Riminucci M, Boyde A. Marrow stromal (Western-Bainton) cells: identification, morphometry, confocal imaging and changes in disease. Bone, 14: 315-320, 1993.
7. Bianco P, Boyde A. Alkaline phosphatase cytochemistry in confocal scanning light microscopy or imaging the bone marrow stroma. Basic Appl Histochem, 33: 17-23, 1989.
8. Bianco P, Costantini M, Dearden LC, Bonucci E. Alkaline phosphatase positive precursors of adipocytes in the human bone marrow. Br J Haematol, 68: 401-403, 1988.
9. Bianco P, Riminucci M, Gronthos S, Robey, PG. Bone marrow stromal stem cells: nature, biology, and potential applications. Stem Cells, 19: 180-192, 2001.
10. Bellahcene A, Albert V, Pollina L, Basolo F, Fishe, LW, Castronovo V. Ectopic expression of bone sialoprotein in human thyroid cancer. Thyroid, 8: 637-641, 1998.
11. Bellahcene A, Castronovo V. Expression of bone matrix proteins in human breast cancer: potential roles in microcalcification formation and in the genesis of bone metastases. Bull Cancer, 84: 17-24, 1997.
12. Robey PG, Bianco P. The cell and molecular biology of bone formation, pp. 199-226. In: *Disorders of Mineral Metabolism.* Coe FL,. Favus MJ, eds, Philadelphia, PA, Lippincott Williams & Wilkin, 2002.
13. Riminucci M, Corsi A, Peris K, Fisher LW, Chimenti S, Bianco P. Coexpression of Bone Sialoprotein (BSP) and the Pivotal Transcriptional Regulator of Osteogenesis, Cbfa1/Runx2, in Malignant Melanoma. Calcif Tissue Int, 2003.
14. Bianco P, Costantini M, Dearden LC, Bonucci E. Expression of tartrate-resistant acid phosphatase in bone marrow macrophages. Basic Appl Histochem, 31: 433-440, 1987.
15. Bianco P, Gehron Robey P. Marrow stromal stem cells. J Clin Invest, 105: 1663-1668, 2000.
16. Friedenstein AJ, Chailakhjan RK, Lalykina KS. The development of fibroblast colonies in monolayer cultures of guinea- pig bone marrow and spleen cells. Cell Tissue Kinet, 3: 393-403, 1970.
17. Gronthos S, Graves SE, Ohta S, Simmons PJ. The STRO-1+ fraction of adult human bone marrow contains the osteogenic precursors. Blood, 84: 4164-4173, 1994.
18. Simmons PJ, Torok-Storb B. Identification of stromal cell precursors in human bone marrow by a novel monoclonal antibody, STRO-1. Blood, 78: 55-62, 1991.
19. Friedenstein AJ, Ivanov-Smolenski AA, Chajlakjan RK, Gorskaya UF, Kuralesova AI, Latzinik NW, Gerasimow UW. Origin of bone marrow stromal mechanocytes in radiochimeras and heterotopic transplants. Exp Hematol, 6: 440-444, 1978.
20. Gronthos S, Zannettino AC, Hay SJ, Shi S, Graves SE, Kortesidis A, Simmons PJ. Molecular and cellular characterisation of highly purified stromal stem cells derived from human bone marrow. J Cell Sci, 116: 1827-1835, 2003.
21. Gronthos S, Simmons PJ, Graves SE, Robey, PG. Integrin-mediated interactions between human bone marrow stromal precursor cells and the extracellular matrix. Bone, 28: 174-181, 2001.

22. Simmons PJ, Masinovsky B, Longenecker BM, Berenson R, Torok-Storb B, Gallatin WM. Vascular cell adhesion molecule-1 expressed by bone marrow stromal cells mediates the binding of hematopoietic progenitor cells. Blood, 80: 388-395, 1992.
23. Shi S, Gronthos S. Perivascular niche of postnatal mesenchymal stem cells in human bone marrow and dental pulp. J Bone Miner Res, 18: 696-704, 2003.
24. Satomura K, Derubeis AR, Fedarko NS, Ibaraki-O'Connor K, Kuznetsov SA, Rowe DW, Young MF, Gehron Robey P. Receptor tyrosine kinase expression in human bone marrow stromal cells. J Cell Physiol, 177: 426-438, 1998.
25. Kuznetsov SA, Krebsbach PH, Satomura K, Kerr J, Riminucci M, Benayahu D, Robey PG. Single-colony derived strains of human marrow stromal fibroblasts form bone after transplantation in vivo. J Bone Miner Res, 12: 1335-1347, 1997.
26. Cooper CR, Pienta KJ. Cell adhesion and chemotaxis in prostate cancer metastasis to bone: a minireview. Prostate Cancer Prostatic Dis, 3: 6-12, 2002.
27. Simmons PJ, Levesque JP, Zannettino AC. Adhesion molecules in haemopoiesis. Baillieres Clin Haematol, 10: 485-505, 1997.
28. Bendall LJ, Gottlieb DJ. CD44 and adhesion of normal and leukemic CD34+ cells to bone marrow stroma. Leuk Lymphoma, 32: 427-439, 1999.
29. Van Driel M, Gunthert U, van Kessel AC, Joling P, Stauder R, Lokhorst HM, Bloem AC. CD44 variant isoforms are involved in plasma cell adhesion to bone marrow stromal cells. Leukemia, 16: 135-143, 2002.
30. Cooper CR, Chay CH, Gendernalik JD, Lee HL, Bhatia J, Taichman RS, McCauley LK, Keller ET, Pienta KJ. Stromal factors involved in prostate carcinoma metastasis to bone. Cancer, 97: 739-747, 2003.
31. Koeneman KS, Yeung F, Chung LW. Osteomimetic properties of prostate cancer cells: a hypothesis supporting the predilection of prostate cancer metastasis and growth in the bone environment. Prostate, 39: 246-261, 1999.
32. Orr FW, Lee J, Duivenvoorden WC, Singh G. Pathophysiologic interactions in skeletal metastasis. Cancer, 88: 2912-2918, 2000.
33. Kitazawa S, Kitazawa R. RANK ligand is a prerequisite for cancer-associated osteolytic lesions. J Pathol, 198: 228-236, 2002.
34. Kakonen SM, Mundy GR. Mechanisms of osteolytic bone metastases in breast carcinoma. Cancer, 97: 834-839, 2003.
35. Friedenstein AJ, Latzinik NW, Grosheva AG, Gorskaya UF. Marrow microenvironment transfer by heterotopic transplantation of freshly isolated and cultured cells in porous sponges. Exp Hematol, 10: 217-227, 1982.
36. Bianco P, Riminucci M, Kuznetsov S, Robey PG. Multipotential cells in the bone marrow stroma: regulation in the context of organ physiology. Crit Rev Eukaryot Gene Expr, 9: 159-173, 1999.
37. Bianco P, Robey PG. Stem cells in tissue engineering. Nature, 414: 118-121, 2001.
38. Bianco P, Kuznetsov SA, Riminucci M, Fisher LW, Spiegel AM, Robey PG. Reproduction of human fibrous dysplasia of bone in immunocompromised mice by transplanted mosaics of normal and Gsalpha-mutated skeletal progenitor cells. J Clin Invest, 101: 1737-1744, 1998.
39. Bianco P, Robey P. Diseases of bone and the stromal cell lineage. J Bone Miner Res, 14: 336-341, 1999.

40. Riminucci M, Collins MT, Corsi A, Boyde A, Murphey MD, Wientroub S, Kuznetsov SA, Cherman N, Robey PG, Bianco P. Gnathodiaphyseal dysplasia: a syndrome of fibro-osseous lesions of jawbones, bone fragility, and long bone bowing. J Bone Miner Res, 16: 1710-1718, 2001.
41. Holmbeck K, Bianco P, Caterina J, Yamada S, Kromer M, Kuznetsov SA, Mankani M, Robey PG, Poole AR, Pidoux I, et al. MT1-MMP-deficient mice develop dwarfism, osteopenia, arthritis, and connective tissue disease due to inadequate collagen turnover. Cell, 99: 81-92, 1999.

80. Penno H, Silfversward CJ, Frost A, Brandstrom H, Nilsson O, Ljunggren O. Osteoprotegerin secretion from prostate cancer is stimulated by cytokines in vitro. Biochem Biophys Res Commun, 293: 451-455, 2002.
81. Holen I, Croucher PI, Handy FC, Eaton CL. Osteoprotegerin (OPG) is a survival factor for human prostate cancer cells. Cancer Res, 62: 1619-1623, 2002.
82. Hofbauer LC, Neubauer A, Heufelder AE. Receptor activator of nuclear factor-kappaB ligand and osteoprotegerin: potential implications for the pathogenesis and treatment of malignant bone diseases. Cancer, 92: 460-470, 2001.
83. Goltzman D. Osteolysis and cancer. J Clin Invest, 107: 1219-1220, 2001.
84. Akatsu T, Murakami T, Ono K, Nishikawa M, Tsuda E, Mochizuki SI, Fujise N, Higashio K, Motoyoshi K, Yamamoto M, Nagata N. Osteoclastogenesis inhibitory factor exhibits hypocalcemic effects in normal mice and in hypercalcemic nude mice carrying tumors associated with humoral hypercalcemia of malignancy. Bone, 23: 495-498, 1998.
85. Capparelli C, Kostenuik PJ, Morony S, Starnes C, Weimann B, Van G, Scully S, Qi M, Lacey DL, Dunstan CR. Osteoprotegerin prevents and reverses hypercalcemia in a murine model of humoral hypercalcemia of malignancy. Cancer Res, 60: 783-787, 2000.
86. Lipton A, Ali SM, Leitzel K, Chinchilli V, Witters L, Engle L, Holloway D, Bekker P, Dunstan CR. Serum osteoprotegerin levels in healthy controls and cancer patients. Clin Cancer Res, 8: 2306-2310, 2002.
87. Honore P, Luger NM, Sabino MA, Schwei MJ, Rogers SD, Mach DB, O'Keefe PF, Ramnaraine ML, Clohisy DR, Mantyh PW. Osteoprotegerin blocks bone cancer-induced skeletal destruction, skeletal pain and pain-related neurochemical reorganization of the spinal cord. Nat Med, 6: 521-528, 2000.
88. Lam J, Takeshita S, Barker JE, Kanagawa O, Ross FP, Teitelbaum SL. TNF-alpha induces osteoclastogenesis by direct stimulation of macrophages exposed to permissive levels of RANK ligand. J Clin Invest, 106: 1481-1488, 2000.
89. Azuma Y, Kaji K, Katogi R, Takeshita S, Kudo A. Tumor necrosis factor-alpha induces differentiation of and bone resorption by osteoclasts. J Biol Chem, 275: 4858-4864, 2000.
90. Kobayashi K, Takahashi N, Jimi E, Udagawa N, Takami M, Kotake S, Nakagawa N, Kinosaki M, Yamaguchi K, Shima N, Yasuda H, Morinaga T, Higashio K, Martin TJ, Suda T. Tumor necrosis factor alpha stimulates osteoclast differentiation by a mechanism independent of the ODF/RANKL-RANK interaction. J Exp Med, 191: 275-286, 2000
91. Kudo O, Fujikawa Y, Itonaga I, Sabokbar A, Torisu T, Athanasou NA. Proinflammatory cytokine (TNFalpha/IL-1alpha) induction of human osteoclast formation. J Pathol,198: 220-227, 2002
92. Kudo O, Sabokbar A, Pocock A, Itonaga I, Fujikawa Y, Athanasou NA. Interleukin-6 and interleukin-11 support human osteoclast formation by a RANKL-independent mechanism. Bone, 32: 1-7, 2003
93. Itonaga I, Sabokbar A, Neale SD, Athanasou NA. 1, 25-Dihydroxyvitamin D3 and prostaglandin E2 act directly on circulating human osteoclast precursors. Biochem Biophys Res Commun, 264: 590-595, 1999.
94. Taylor PC. Anti-TNFα therapy for rheumatoid arthritis: an update. Intern Med, 42: 15-20, 2003.
95. Teti A, Migliacero S, Baron R. The role of alpha v beta 3 integrin in the development of osteolytic bone metastases: a pharmacological target for alternative therapy. Calcif Tissue Int, 71: 293-299, 2002.

Chapter 7

THE MALIGNANT HIERARCHY IN MULTIPLE MYELOMA: RELATIONSHIPS BETWEEN MALIGNANT CELLS AND BONE DISEASE

Linda M. Pilarski, Tony Reiman, Patrick M. Pilarski, F. William Orr and Andrew R. Belch
University of Alberta and Cross Cancer Institute, and University of Manitoba, Alberta, Canada

1. INTRODUCTION

Multiple myeloma (MM) is an incurable cancer of the bone marrow (BM), with survival of 3-4 years. MM accounts for 1% of all cancers, and 19% of deaths from hematological malignancies. It is characterized by monoclonal immunoglobulin (mIg) in the blood, lytic bone lesions, and monoclonal plasma cells in the BM. These plasma cells are responsible for most symptoms of MM, but considerable work confirms that the MM clone also includes earlier stage B lymphocytes. The MM clone is characterized by an immunoglobulin variable region gene rearrangement (IgH VDJ), termed "clonotypic". The IgH VDJ rearrangement that defines the MM clone in each patient is unique, thus providing an unequivocal molecular signature for MM cells regardless of, for example, genetic abnormalities, phenotype, morphology or physical location. Although the phenotypic properties of the MM clone are altered as the disease progresses and genetic heterogeneity increases, the clonotypic IgH VDJ signature remains constant, exhibiting rigid intraclonal homogeneity of sequence (1-3). With the exception of plasma cells, the distribution of the myeloma clone *in situ*, and its relationship to bone lesions within the BM is largely unknown. Because it is at best difficult, and at worst impossible to morphologically or

G. Singh and W. Orr (eds.), Bone Metastasis and Molecular Mechanisms, 109-138.

phenotypically distinguish the earlier stage members of the MM clone from normal B lineage cells, detection of the IgH VDJ MM signature is essential as the distinguishing characteristic of individual MM cells participating in the apparently synergistic relationship between bone and malignancy.

The MM clone is highly heterogeneous, including multiple differentiation stages (Figure 1 A, B). The originating events and the subpopulations that promote bone destruction and osteoclast activity *in vivo* are unknown. Although provocative reports exist, there has been no characterization of the architecture of the MM clone *in situ* as it relates to physical relationships between subpopulations of MM cells and developing bone lesions. The widely applied reductionist approach involving analysis of cellular interactions *in vitro*, particularly those involving bone metabolism, must be extended to an *in vivo* context, to analyze the impact of therapy on these bone/malignancy inter-relationships. This is particularly true for agents such as bisphosphonates, which appear to have a profound impact on MM patients and possibly on the MM clone as well. Although nearly all MM patients are treated with bisphosphonates, there have as yet been no longitudinal studies in patients to define the characteristics of bone metabolism and tumor architecture during treatment with chemotherapy plus bisphosphonates *in vivo*. A careful analysis of bone disease in MM may lead to improved treatment options for MM patients by enabling the development of novel therapies to disrupt the synergistic cycle of tumor/bone interactions, halt bone damage and improve survival for patients with this deadly cancer.

Some MM patients are diagnosed at very early, largely asymptomatic stages of disease; these are termed indolent or smoldering MM and are usually left untreated until the disease progresses to more aggressive stages. Many patients with overt MM respond to melphalan/prednisone or vincristine/adriamycin/dexamethasone (VAD), but nearly all relapse and become refractory to treatment (4, 5). Autologous stem cell transplants achieve some complete remissions and prolong survival (6-11), but are not curative. Allogeneic transplantation has a high treatment-related mortality and few patients are eligible (10, 12). MM may arise through progressive acquisition of genetic abnormalities (13-15), and is characterized by complex chromosomal abnormalities (16). Although MM pathology is thought to result from plasma cells, no correlation is detectable between decrement in serum mIg or plasma cell kill after conventional chemotherapy and patient survival (17, 18). A modest increase in survival is found after cytoreduction and autologous transplantation (6). Generative potential within the MM clone may derive from less differentiated components.

(40). The heterogeneity seen among *ex-vivo* clonotypic B cells suggests an *in vivo* hierarchy of sequentially related differentiation stages (Figure 1). The extent to which these early stage clonotypic cells inhabit the BM, participate in the generation of plasma cells and contribute to bone lesions remains to be addressed. It is important to emphasize that the early stage members of the MM clone are morphologically "cryptic" in that their physical appearance and phenotypic profiles are largely normal, preventing their identification using morphological criteria as "morphologically abnormal" cells. Only their expression of the clonotypic IgH VDJ signature confirms their relationship within the malignant clone.

2. BONE DISEASE IN MM

Although *ex-vivo* analysis of MM has provided valuable insights into the disease process, fundamentally, MM is a disease of the BM. MM pathology occurs in the BM. It is likely that generative phases of disease are also BM-localized, and that physical relationships between MM components and the cells responsible for bone metabolism are biologically important. Bone disease is a central pathological complication of MM. Most patients have characteristic lytic bone lesions in trabecular bone, osteoporosis is common, histomorphometry shows frequent trabecular damage, and fracturing of fragile bone is frequent. Osteoclasts are present in abnormal numbers lining regions of damaged bone, and the most commonly held view is that factors elaborated by MM plasma cells are responsible for activation of osteoclast differentiation and bone resorbing activity. Osteoblast function has been less extensively characterized. Osteoblast recruitment was actually increased in MM as compared to monoclonal gammopathy of undetermined significance (MGUS), but appeared to be significantly reduced in patients with overt MM as compared to those with early MM (68). However this was coupled with increased formation of new osteoclasts and increased bone resorption. As noted by Bataille and colleagues (68), factors from the MM clone may led to increased osteoblast function, which in turn may further stimulate the MM clone through production of growth factors such as IL-6, leading to increased MM-promoted osteoclastic activity. Thus MM appears to be characterized by interlinked and synergistic pathways of tumor growth and bone erosion. It is widely believed that all of these effects are mediated by the end stage malignant plasma cells that inhabit the bone marrow in MM. Here, we argue that earlier members of the MM hierarchy contribute to the maintenance of MM bone lesions when the cancer is in minimal stages, and that the MM clone may directly contribute to the bone erosion that characterizes the disease. This view of MM pathology is supported by observations such as those of Rondelli and colleagues who described the appearance of new bone lesions in patients who have achieved complete remission after transplant (69). Osteoclasts are known to arise from monocytoid progenitors. We speculate that circulating monocytoid MM B cells, shown to be clonotypic using single cell RT-PCR analysis of IgH transcripts, may function as osteoclastic progenitors, thus contributing in a direct fashion to MM bone damage. This is supported by known links between B cells and macrophages (70). If this view is correct, it means that the MM hierarchy comprises two distinct but clonally related arms, one that gives rise to MM plasma cells and their associated pathological complications, and one that leads directly to osteoclast activity and bone erosion.

In MM, analysis of the BM has been limited by the inability to distinguish clonotypic from non-clonotypic populations of cells *in situ*. Although the patterns of plasma cell localization have been well characterized in MM at diagnosis, there has been little or no analysis of BM architecture, cell-cell interactions, or the precise distribution of the MM clone within the BM. For other cancers (e.g., breast and prostate) some evidence exists to suggest that tumor cells themselves have bone resorbing activity (71-73). As indicated above, based on a variety of suggestive observations, malignant components of the MM clone may also have direct bone resorbing activity, particularly during stages of minimal disease. The need to design more effective modes of therapy demands that MM/bone interactions be more extensively characterized *in situ*.

2.1 MM Bone Disease

In complete skeletons from two persons clinically diagnosed with MM while still alive, lytic bone lesions were seen as sharply defined spheroid areas, having smooth borders and internal surfaces with no evidence of new bone formation (74). MM lesions are distinctive as compared to those of metastatic carcinoma (74). Osteoclasts are multinuclear, macrophage-like hematopoietic cells that destroy bone. Overall, osteoclast numbers are increased only in bone resorption lacunae closely proximate to plasma cells (75), with a high correlation between numbers of plasma cells and osteoclasts (76). Of interest, patients with dense infiltrates of plasma cells often have few bone lesions, suggesting the importance of factors other than plasma cells (77, Belch, unpublished).

For many patients, plasma cell infiltration is accompanied by osteolytic lesions, causing fractures and bone pain. In normal BM, plasma cells are associated with vascular structures (sinusoids, venules and around capillaries). In early MM, plasma cells are loosely dispersed between fat and hematopoietic cells. In later stages, plasma cells form sheets that are distant from vascular structures (78). Although chemotherapy reduces the plasma cell mass, it does not improve histological bone lesions in areas where plasma cells remain detectable (79), even though skeletal invasion by plasma cells is decreased. For a subset of MGUS, increased bone resorption in the vicinity of plasma cells suggested ongoing progression to MM (75). Although one study using bone histomorphometry has found few differences between untreated or chemotherapy-treated patients having heavy infiltration with plasma cells (79), there are no published histological analyses of MM bone lesions over time or as a function of therapy-induced reductions in plasma cell infiltration.

Interestingly, a high bone mineral density (BMD) has been found in the forearm (which lacks marrow), although the femoral neck and lumbar spine had low BMD (80), consistent with the view that marrow-localized cells influence the reduced BMD of MM patients. No correlation was found between BMD and presence or extent of lytic lesions (80). In contrast, serum paraprotein and % plasma cells were the most important predictors of femoral neck bone loss (81). Another study found that responders to therapy, and hence patients getting high-dose therapy, tend to do better in the context of changes in bone density than nonresponders/patients on conventional chemotherapy (82).

The inability to reverse bone damage and the persistence of bone lesions, even in stages of minimal disease, suggests that clinically cryptic components of the MM clone persist despite therapy and perpetuate dysregulated bone metabolism. Our observations that bone lesions are readily detectable in xenografted mice having few or no detectable plasma cells suggests that early stage MM cells themselves may have the ability to dysregulate bone metabolism (53, 63, 64). The evidence cited above supports the hypothesis that early stage B lineage MM cells interact with bone and contribute to bone lesions, as well as providing compelling justification for analysis of early stage members of the MM clone and their direct/indirect relationships to bone damage in MM.

2.2 Lymphoid Cells and Bone Lesions

Although lymphoid cells appear to influence bone pathology, there are no published studies to characterize the potential influence of lymphoid members of the MM clone on bone pathology. The fairly limited number of studies that have identified plasma cells in proximity to osteoclasts and bone lesions did not analyze lymphocytes that may have also been proximate, and in any case would have lacked the tools to determine whether or not any proximate lymphocytes were components of the MM clone. Reports of B cell malignancies mimicking the bone disease found in MM indicate that B cells can promote lytic bone lesions (83). Provocatively, in BM with a nodular distribution of plasma cells, lymphocytes were found at the center of nodules, with mature plasma cells located in the marginal regions (78). In MM, frequent lymphoid *nodules* were associated with fewer lytic bone lesions and better prognosis (78, 84), but MM patients with diffuse lymphocytosis in BM had a shorter survival (78). Post transplant/donor lymphocyte infusion, an MM patient was found to develop new bone lesions despite the apparent absence of plasma cells or serum M protein (69). Anecdotal macroscopic observations indicate that bone lesions may fail to heal when disease enters remission.

Bone lesions were found in mice xengrafted with clonotypic lymphoid cells or with hematopoietic cells, having little, if any, plasma cell engraftment within the murine BM (63, 64) suggesting a role for lymphoid cells in the generation of bone lesions. Our hypothesis is that bone lesions persist despite successful chemotherapy because clonotypic MM B cells remain (23, 25, 41, 42) and continue to promote bone disease. The literature is conflicting in assessing healing of bone lesions in MM (77, 80-82, 85, 86). Some reports indicate that bones can and do heal in association with response to therapy, with an increase in bone mineral density as measured by X-ray, CT or MRI (77, 80, 82, 86), although bone lesions do not improve (85). However, the prognostic significance of this is unclear, with two groups showing that patients having normal X-rays or whose lesions heal on X-ray do worse (87, 88), perhaps because their disease is more diffuse, and two concluding that patients do better if the lesions heal (86, 89). Diamond et al. found that bone mineral density decreased over the course of conventional chemotherapy (81). Our local experience is that bone lesions can improve but that the improvement tends to be modest (TR, unpublished); usually there is no improvement seen when repeat x-rays are performed. Morphometric analysis of patients treated with chemotherapy suggest a lack of healing at the microscopic level (79). The relationship to the MM clone of lymphocytes that are proximal to regions of bone damage has not been examined, nor have the beneficial effects of bisphosphonates been correlated with a possible impact on lymphocytic members of the MM clone.

3. LYTIC BONE LESIONS IN MM PATIENTS

Although numerous studies have characterized the cells involved in bone metabolism *in vitro* or in animal models, very little, if any, work has analyzed the bone changes *in vivo* that accompany human MM as the disease waxes and wanes, ultimately progressing to extensive bone damage and death. Bone damage is directly responsible for the adverse quality of life for MM patients and is a primary symptom of the disease.

Two potent intravenous bisphosphonates, pamidronate or zoledronic acid are most frequently used to reduce skeletal related adverse events in nearly all MM patients (90). Bisphosphonates adsorb to bone mineral and inhibit bone resorption by inhibiting osteoclast activity (91, 92). They appear to break the cycle of osteoclast bone destruction promoted by the MM clone, and significantly reduce bone fractures, but the mechanisms of action are far from clear. Evidence is accumulating to suggest that they act by inhibiting cytokines (93-95), and may alter micro-environmental interactions in MM (91). Finally, bisphosphonates may directly target the MM clone as well as inhibiting osteoclast activity (96). Patients not receiving bisphosphonates continue to lose bone during chemotherapy, probably in part due to the steroid therapy, whereas patients receiving bisphosphonates tend to gain in bone density (80, 97). However there was also a lack of correlation between bone density and the presence/extent of lytic lesions. Oral risendronate was shown to incease spinal bone mineral density, decrease serum markers of bone resorption, normalize bone turnover, and reduce histomorphometric measures of bone loss (77).

Some patients with extensive plasma cell infiltration lack detectable bone lesions, contrary to the expectation that factors from plasma cells stimulate osteoclast activity. Further, even though patients can enter "complete remissions" after autologous transplant, macroscopically detected bone lesions often do not heal, an unexpected observation if the dogma that plasma cells cause bone disease is correct, because transplant occurs at stages of minimal disease and plasma cell levels are severely depleted immediately post-transplant. These and other anecdotal observations suggest that bone pathology can be mediated through malignant MM components other than plasma cells. Analysis of human disease cannot adequately be described through analysis of model systems. A precise evaluation of the bone changes in MM and the cells responsible has to be founded on a thorough histomorphometric longitudinal analysis of bone pathology that records quantitative characteristics of bone damage at diagnosis, and as disease is treated, responds and relapses.

3.1 Histomorphometric Analysis of Bone in MM

Histomorphometry generates quantitative measures of bone volume, mineralization, and rates of remodeling that can be correlated directly with definition of molecular phenotypes of cells in the local bone microenvironment. Bone morphometry has been used extensively to define the pathophysiology of metabolic bone diseases, e.g., osteoporosis, with infrequent IgM expression ($p<0.0001$). In a multivariate analysis, persistent clonotypic IgM expression in the blood correlated independently with poor survival ($p=0.01$). In NOD SCID mice, xenografted MM cells expressed clinical and non-clinical post-switch clonotypic isotypes. Xenografted cells expressing clonotypic IgM were clonogenic and appeared to be self-renewing in murine BM (40). We speculate that myeloma may originate from a clonotypic IgM precursor cell that undergoes persistent isotype switching throughout the disease, leading to terminal plasma cell differentiation in the BM and perhaps initiating bone disease.

4.3 Circulating MM Cells Generate MM Bone Disease on Xenotransplant

The myelomagenic capacity of clonotypic MM cells during aggressive disease and in stages of minimal disease, defined by G-CSF mobilized autografts, were tested by xenotransplant (53). Intra-cardiac (IC) injection of immunodeficient NOD SCID mice with peripheral cells from 5 patients having aggressive myeloma led to lytic bone lesions, human Ig in the serum, human plasma cells and a high frequency of clonotypic cells in the murine BM. Intra-osseous (IO) injection of *ex vivo* MM cells directly into the murine sternal BM led to lytic bone lesions (Figure 2), BM plasma cells and a high frequency of clonotypic cells in the femoral BM. This indicates the spread of MM from the primary injection site to distant BM locations and subsequent initiation of macroscopically detectable bone damage.

Using a cellular limiting dilution PCR assay to quantify clonotypic B lineage cells, we confirmed that peripheral MM cells home to murine BM. The MM progenitor undergoes self-renewal in murine BM, as demonstrated by the transfer of human MM to a secondary recipient mouse. To obtain hematopoietic stem cells for autologous transplants, patients are treated with cyclophosphamide and G-CSF (a growth factor), a procedure termed mobilization. Mobilization causes stem cells to leave the BM and accumulate in the blood where they are harvested, cryopreserved and eventually reinfused after high dose chemotherapy. Mobilized blood stem cell autografts from 6/7 MM patients, taken at the time of mobilization or after cryopreservation, included MM progenitors as identified by engraftment of clonotypic cells and/or lytic bone disease in mice. This indicates that MM progenitors are mobilized into the blood, and are present even during stages of minimal disease. Such residual cells are likely to contribute to post-transplant relapse and to mediate persistent bone disease. The ability of mobilized autografts to generate MM after xenotransplantation implies that such progenitors are also myelomagenic when reinfused to patients, and suggests the need for an effective purging strategy prior to transplant. We speculate that *in vivo*, these same MM cells home to, and colonize patient BM, thus perpetuating the cycle of homing to trabecular bone and bone damage that characterizes MM *in vivo*.

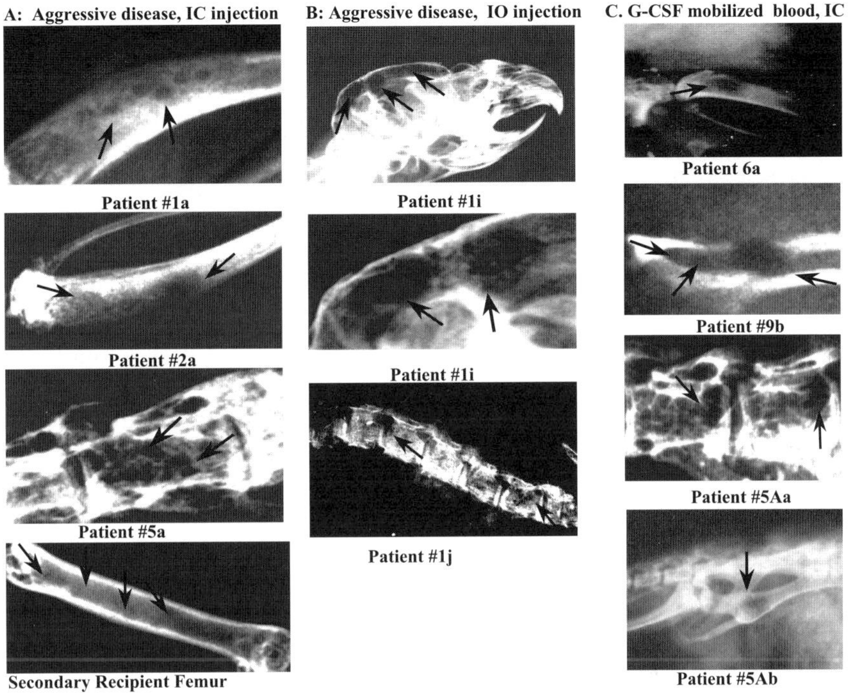

Figure 2. Lytic bone lesions in xenografted mice. IC - intracArdiac injection, IO - intraosseus injection. Patients listed as having aggressive disease had circulating plasma cells. Patients from whom G-CSF mobilized blood autografts were obtained were in minimal disease. Pilarski et al. Myeloma progenitors in the blood of patients with aggressive or minimal disease: Engraftment and self-renewal of primary human myeloma in the bone marrow of NOD SCID mice. Blood 95:1056-1065, 2000. Copyright American Society of Hematology, used with permission.

4.4 MM B Lymphocytes Generate Lytic Bone Disease in Xenografted Mice

Although MM plasma cells express CD138 (syndecan-1), clonotypic myeloma B cells are $CD19^{+}138^{-}$ in all patients tested. Using single cell RT-PCR and PCR, we showed that aggressive circulating lymphoblasts from an MM patient who developed Burkitt's-like lymphoblastoid leukemia were all clonotypic with an IgH VDJ sequence *identical* to that of autologous plasma cells at diagnosis (64). Flow cytometric analysis showed leukemic B cells were $CD19^+$ 138^-. For both the myeloma and the leukemic phases of the disease, the clinical clonotypic isotype was IgA. Analysis of IgH transcripts indicates MM clonal dominance over normal components of the immune system at diagnosis and prior to terminal Burkitt's lymphoma-like leukemic disease. $CD138^-$ leukemic B cells were xenografted to irradiated NOD SCID mice via intra-cardiac injection. At 3-4 months post-engraftment, lytic bone lesions and clonotypic cells were detected in the BM of engrafted mice (64). Although a subset of human cells in the murine BM expressed CD138, a marker largely absent from *ex vivo* leukemic cells, the expression of CD45, CD19 and CD20 confirmed that engrafting cells were late stage B-cells rather than plasma cells. Thus, leukemic B-cells colonize the murine BM in a xenograft model, and disrupt normal bone metabolism leading to lytic bone lesions. This supports the hypothesis that clonotypic MM B-cells are reservoirs of disease that persist throughout therapy and play a significant role in dysregulated bone metabolism and bone damage. It also provides strong justification for the hypothesis that MM B cells are direct and/or indirect contributors to the cycle of bone homing and bone destruction in MM.

4.5 Xenografted Progenitor-like MM Cells Give Rise to Clonotypic MM Cells and Lytic Bone Lesions

The identity of MM precursor(s) is unknown, and the contributions to MM pathology of early stage components of the MM clone remain unclear. To address this question, the myelomagenic capabilities and contributions to lytic bone disease of CD34-enriched autografts were determined (63). Hematopoietic progenitor fractions from fresh or cryopreserved G-CSF mobilized blood from MM patients were obtained by sorting or enrichment, followed by RT-PCR analysis of clonotypic transcripts and/or their ability to transfer myeloma to immunodeficient mice. Highly purified $CD34^+$ progenitors from G-CSF mobilized blood of myeloma patients include on average, 24% clonotypic MM cells. $CD34^+$ progenitors also include 31% DNA aneuploid cells.

For 6/6 MM patients, enriched progenitors were myelomagenic on xenograft analysis, as measured by engraftment of clonotypic cells and/or the development of lytic bone lesions. The majority of mice (73%, range 60-100%) engrafted with enriched progenitors had lytic lesions in the skull, spine, pelvis and/or tibia. Bone lesions were found at distant locations in mice injected intra-sternally, further confirming the spread of disease that had originated from the enriched progenitors. No lesions were detected in irradiated control mice that had not received enriched progenitors. The presence of bone lesions at distant skeletal locations confirms dissemination of myelomagenic cells throughout the skeleton, the preferential homing to bone sites and the generation of bone lesions either directly or indirectly from early stage, resting lymphocytes with clonotypic IgH VDJ.

The involved cells are likely to be post germinal center, memory B cells, given that clonotypic transcripts detected in sorted or enriched progenitor populations appear to be predominantly post-switch IgG or IgA cells with a somatically mutated IgH VDJ clonotypic sequence identical to that of autologous plasma cells. Unlike mice xenografted with leukemic plasma cells (53, 64), the lesions in mice injected with enriched progenitor fractions were less pronounced and clonotypic transcripts were less frequent (63). This may reflect different degrees of differentiation for MM precursors among leukemic plasma cells and those among earlier stage B cells, since end stage plasma cells have considerably higher levels of Ig and Ig transcripts which are more readily detected in our assays. Within the 1-3 month window evaluated here, MM precursors present among CD34-enriched progenitors may not complete differentiation to plasma cell stages, resulting in engrafted MM cells with lower transcript copy numbers.

These observations implicate early stage MM components in the generation of lytic bone disease. For many mice, lytic bone lesions were readily detectable even though clonotypic transcripts were below our levels of detection. This suggests that bone lesions and/or altered bone metabolism was induced in the absence of differentiation by MM progenitors to end stage plasma cells. By extrapolation, this work is supportive of a role for malignant lymphocytes in the generation of bone disease in MM, providing further justification for the hypothesis that MM B lymphocytes home to bone, disrupt normal bone metabolism and are significant participants in MM bone pathology.

Both plasma cells and lymphocytes have been reported to have prognostic significance in BM biopsies at diagnosis (78, 84). Lymphoid nodules are detectable in MM BM (78, 84), lymphocytic infiltrates persist after high dose chemotherapy (116), and plasma cell nodules have centrally located lymphocytes (78). Together with the evidence cited above, it seems possible that lymphocytes contribute to early stages of bone disease, as identified histologically, while plasma cells may be required to stimulate massive bone destruction that leads to lytic bone lesions identified macroscopically. It is unknown whether the lack of new bone synthesis in MM represents a systemic defect in osteoblast function, or if it represents a localized uncoupling of bone loss and gain caused by proximity to malignant cells.

5. FUNCTIONAL PROPERTIES OF LYMPHOCYTIC CELLS IN BM LESIONS

Although the evidence from our work and that of others clearly indicates that the MM clone includes a hierarchy of B lineage cells, the extent to which any or all of these cell types serve as generative reservoirs of human disease *in situ* remains ambiguous. The early members of the MM clone appear to be drug resistant components that persist throughout conventional and high dose chemotherapy. Although novel biologically based therapies such as thalidomide are proving very effective in MM, patients still relapse, indicative of drug resistant components despite achieving complete remission (as defined by undetectable levels of mIg). Drug-resistant B cell members of the MM hierarchy may be significant components of the process that ultimately leads to relapse. However as indicated above, it appears that multiple components of the MM clone have the ability to transfer disease and/or correlate with reduced survival. Taken together, work by ourselves and others indicates that progenitor function in MM occurs at several levels, and must be evaluated in terms of an ability to generate as progeny the plasma cells that contribute to bone pathology, and ultimately to patient death.

5.1 Plasma Cells

It is widely believed that the primary generative components of MM are the BM-localized plasma cells that cause symptoms and pathology, including bone disease, of MM. No matter which B cell maturation stages harbor progenitor function and which lead to osteoclastic bone resorption, the ultimate mediators of MM are likely to be BM plasma cells. For example, early stage MM cells may mediate osteoclast generation during stages of minimal disease while in aggressive disease the extensive plasma cell infiltration may stimulate clonally normal osteoclastic activity. Hypothetically, since plasma cells have such extensive ability to mediate disease pathology, if they are able to undergo even a minimal number of generative cycles, they will be detected as "myelomagenic" in model systems and in patients. We predict that plasma cells with progenitor function will rapidly generate detectable disease because they have already terminally differentiated to the pathological stage (as diagrammed in Figure 3). This prediction appears to be supported in both a Hu-SCID model in which BM plasma cells are injected directly into a human fetal bone implant under the kidney capsule of an immmunodeficient mouse (117, 118), and in our own work injecting leukemic plasma cells to NOD SCID mice (53). In both cases, the abundant plasma cells appear to rapidly engraft and cause bone lesions. However, this cannot be a complete picture since in patients, the number of plasma cells in BM autografts does not appear to correlate with survival (4). In all of these examples where plasma cells have apparent progenitor function, it seems likely that aggressive plasma cell progeny cause death before any impact of therapy targeting/depleting earlier stage progenitors could be detected.

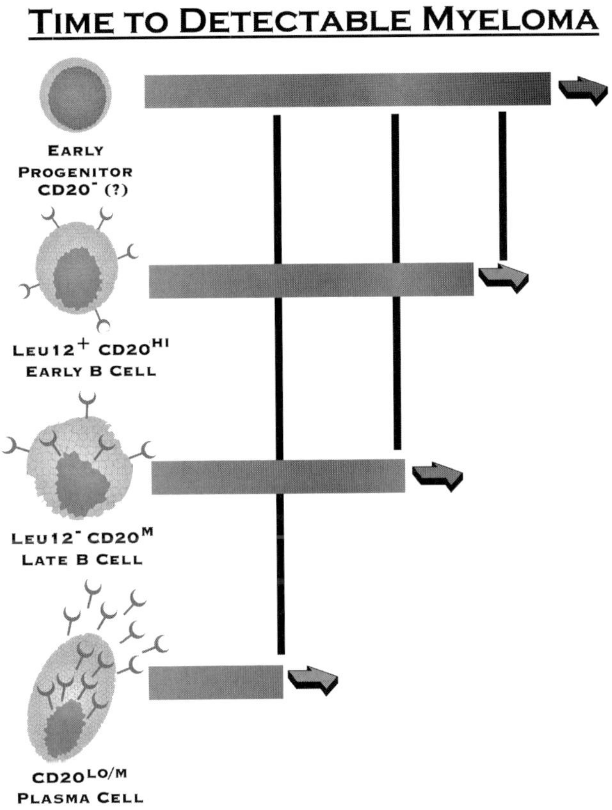

Figure 3. Heterogeneity in MM progenitor cells. The time to detectable disease depends upon the maturation stage of the progenitor fraction of MM cells. Early stage progenitors are predicted to exhibit a prolonged delay before disease becomes detectable, and to have extensive self renewal capabilities. Late stage progenitors are predicted to lead to rapid symptomatic disease, and to have quite limited self renewal capability. Since the plasma cell pool is predicted to be readily replenished by early stage progenitors, depletion of late stage progenitors is likely to be reversed by drug resistant earlier stage progenitors. Thus therapeutic attack must be targeted to both early and late stage disease components.

5.2 Mature B Cells

G-CSF mobilized blood from patients in minimal disease xenografted human MM to NOD SCID mice (53). For 9/9 mobilized blood preparations, <0.01% plasma cells were detected, but $CD19^{+}$ B cells were readily detectable by their clonotypic transcripts (63). For 6/7 patients tested, mobilized blood engrafted murine BM, as detected by clonotypic transcripts and bone lesions (53). Interestingly, mice xenografted with mobilized blood autografts had readily detectable bone lesions on X-ray, despite the absence of detectable plasma cells in their marrow. The frequency of mice with detectable clonotypic transcripts was also lower suggesting that differentiation had not yet reached abundant plasma cell stages, at which time transcript copy numbers would be extremely high and easily detectable. This work suggests the presence of a mature B cell progenitor stage, with the ability to cause disease, but by virtue of their mature B cell stage, a delayed ability to generate end stage plasma cells relative to progenitor-competent plasma cells (Figure 3). This is borne out by the analysis of leukemic B cells that developed in a MM patient (64). These circulating, clonotypic B cells were able to engraft BM and generate lytic bone lesions in the absence of visible symptoms or detectable plasma cell progeny. For the normal immune system, the concept that earlier progenitors require a longer time to generate end stage effector cells is widely held and supported by immunological experiments (119-121).

Pre-switch MM cells also engraft immunodeficient mice (40), leading to pre-switch clonotypic cells in murine BM, but the extent to which these cells contributed to bone lesions in such mice could not be evaluated. However, for xenografted circulating cells from one patient, the *only* clonotypic transcripts detected in BM and spleen were of the IgM isotype (Figure 4). All three xenografted mice had detectable osteolytic lesions, suggesting these originated from engraftment of pre-switch MM B cells derived from the peripheral blood xenograft. In contrast, all clonotypic isotypes were detected within vertebral masses that arose in these mice (Figure 4).

A large concentration of human MM cells may be a prerequisite for the expression of post-switch isotypes (as detected in the vertebral masses). The absence of post-switch clonotypic isotypes in lymphoid tissues may reflect a lesser degree of clonal expansion by pre-switch MM precursors, as compared to the macroscopically greater expansion in the vertebral tumor masses, consistent with observations of Hodgkin and co-workers showing that isotype switching increases with the number of clonal divisions (122). As well, a high concentration of MM cells may be needed to maintain and/or to generate cells of post-switch clonotypic isotypes, perhaps reflecting production of human cytokines and/or a requirement for cellular interactions.

Direct evidence that pre-switch progenitors may have a strong influence on MM progression comes from our longitudinal analysis (40) which showed a strong correlation between persistent, and thus drug-resistant, pre-switch MM cells and reduced survival ($p<0.0001$). Thus in patients, where the pre-switch MM cells have a prolonged time in which to undergo clonal expansion and differentiation to plasma cell stages, a clinical impact is detected. In this context, the relationship between pre-switch MM cells and bone disease is unknown. However the data of Figure 3 suggests they may cause bone lesions. This reinforces the idea that evaluation of progenitor function in MM must take into account the parameters of time and maturation stage.

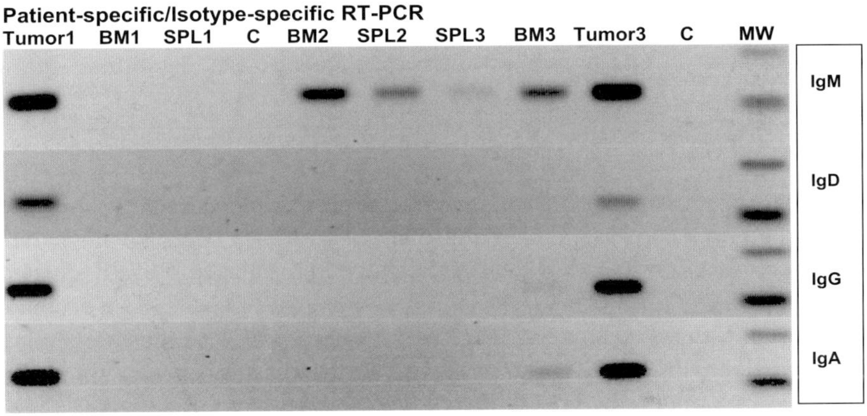

Figure 4. Clonotypic IgM transcripts in spleen and BM of mice xenografted with PBMC from a relapsed MM patient. Three xenografted mice developed visible symptoms and were sacrificed at about 3 months post-engraftment. Large vertebral masses were found in all three mice. T- tumor vertebral mass, BM- bone marrow, Spl- spleen, C-PCR control lanes. Nested PCR used VHLeader/constant region primers followed by CDR2/CDR3 patient-specific primers (22).

5.3 CD19$^-$ MM Progenitors

We have shown by a variety of measures that CD34$^+$ hematopoietic progenitor populations include clonotypic MM cells, but lack detectable plasma cells (63). These CD34-enriched fractions composed of normal progenitors and MM cells engraft MM clonotypic transcripts to NOD SCID BM and lead to lytic bone lesions. Since CD19 mAb is included in the cocktail of antibodies used to deplete lineage committed cells, the MM progenitors being detected here appear to lack CD19 but are clearly mature memory B cells by virtue of a somatically mutated IgH VDJ in the inoculated cells and in their progeny in the engrafted mice. These engrafted mice did not exhibit visible disease symptoms and clonotypic transcripts were detectable in only 18% of mice suggesting that their progeny were not plasma cells but rather earlier stage cells with low transcript copy numbers. The dilemma in MM, illustrated in Figure 3, is that if only plasma cells are eradicated, the MM B cell progenitors described above will still mediate bone disease and will eventually restore the plasma cell component leading to re-emergence of disease, continuation of bone erosion and relapse. If only the early stage progenitors are eradicated, the plasma cells remaining in the patient will lead to relapse and death. This means that for MM, combination therapeutic strategies designed to target multiple components of the MM clone will be required to halt the progression of the MM clone and improve patient survival.

5.4 Myeloma and Bone Metabolism

A variety of cytokines control bone metabolism, with osteoblasts creating new bone and osteoclasts destroying bone (114, 123). The final mediators are osteoprotegerin-ligand [OPGL, a tumor necrosis factor (TNF)-related cytokine], RANK, the cell surface receptor for OPGL, and OPG a secreted TNF receptor family member (124). OPG sequesters OPGL, thus preventing its interaction with RANK, to down-regulate osteoclast differentiation (125). Thus, osteoclastogenesis is inhibited by OPG and promoted by OPGL (124, 126). OPG functions as an inhibitor of osteolytic bone disease in an animal model of MM (127). OPGL (RANKL) is detectable as a surface membrane receptor on normal B cells (128) and MM plasma cells (129). In this context it is interesting that MM B cells bind OPG -FITC (a recombinant OPG lacking the heparin binding domain) (AJ Szczepek and LM Pilarski, unpublished), suggesting that they may be stimulated in some way through binding of OPG and may play a significant role in disordered bone metabolism. Other key cytokines involved in osteoclastogenesis are IL-6 and colony-stimulating factor-1 (CSF-1) (114). Plasma cells may exacerbate this process by syndecan-1 mediated sequestering of OPG (92), and/or production of OPGL, thus increasing the active concentrations of OPGL. Although controversial, several groups have detected RANKL on myeloma plasma cells (129, 130). Serum OPG is reduced in MM patients having lytic bone disease (131-133), again suggesting an intimate relationship between the MM clone and bone disease. MM B lymphocytes constitutively express IL-6 and IL-6R (66), as well as expressing CSF-1 and CSF-1R (LMP, unpublished), suggesting they may play an important role in osteoclastogenesis in the BM. Possibilities are a) they themselves are osteoclast progenitors, as predicted by reference (134), under autocrine growth promotion, or b) they produce paracrine factors that stimulate osteoclast differentiation.

It has been speculated that members of the MM clone may differentiate to osteoclasts (134). Our own work raises the possibility that MM clonotypic B cells, which have monocytoid properties and morphology, may differentiate to osteoclasts or perhaps themselves directly participate in bone resorption. This notion is supported by work showing that MM PBMC include unidentified osteoclast precursors that give rise *in vitro* to osteoclasts with bone resorbing capability (135). Provocatively, CD56 (NCAM) was strongly expressed by ostoclasts and osteoblasts, but only in MM with lytic bone lesions did $CD138^+$ plasma cells coexpress $CD56^{hi}$ (lymphocytes were not evaluated in this study) (136), suggesting that homophilic binding between these cells, mediated by CD56, was important for both decreased bone formation and increased bone resorption. In this context, it may be significant that high levels of CD56 are also expressed by MM B cells (25), which have the potential for autocrine secretion of osteoclastogenic factors that may also inhibit osteoblast function (66). Finally, recent work shows that early stage normal B cells have the potential to differentiate into osteoclasts (128), lending support to the view that malignant B cells may retain this capability and raising the possibility that the clonotypic IgM-expressing MM B cells described above (40) may influence survival via an impact on bone metabolism. The view that MM B lymphocytes may be directly responsible for bone destruction is supported by our xenograft analysis of human MM (53, 64). Lytic bone lesions were detected in mice xenografted with early stage human cells that had little, if any, plasma cell infiltration in the murine BM (53, 63, 64), suggestive of a role for lymphocytic members of the MM clone in this process.

6. CONCLUSIONS

Although the idea that MM cells themselves may directly contribute to bone damage in MM, as opposed to indirectly through stimulation of normal osteoclastogenesis, challenges current dogma regarding the pathology of MM, it is important to test this hypothesis. A central issue is to determine the extent to which, if any, MM cells themselves contribute directly to bone damage since this is such a significant aspect of MM pathology. The pathological effects of monocytoid, clonotypic B cells in MM are unclear, but they have many of the properties thought to characterize osteoclast progenitors, including a cytokine profile consistent with autocrine

61. Pilarski LM, Yatscoff RW, Murphy G, Belch AR. Drug resistance in multiple myeloma: Cyclosporin analogues and metabolites as chemosensitizers. Leukemia, 12: 505-509, 1998.
62. Treon SP, Mollick JA, Urashima M, Teoh G, Chauhan D, Ogata A, Raje N, Hilgers JM, Nadler L, Belch AR, et al. Muc-1 core protein is expressed on multiple myeloma cells and is induced by dexamethasone. Blood, 93: 1287-1298, 1999.
63. Pilarski LM, Belch AR. Clonotypic Myeloma Cells Able to Xenograft Myeloma to NOD SCID mice are Detectable Among $CD34^+$ Hematopoietic Progenitors. Clin Cancer Res, 8: 3198-3204, 2002.
64. Pilarski LM, Seeberger K, Keats JJ, Taylor BJ, Coupland RW, Belch AR. Leukemic B cells clonally identical to myeloma plasma cells are myelomagenic in NOD SCID mice. Exp Hematol, 30: 221-228, 2002.
65. Straka C, Mitterer M, Oduncu F, Drexler E, Schnabel B, Suttmann I, Bleicher R, Langenmayer I, Buhlmann H, Auchter K, et al. Immunomagnetic ex vivo B cell purging in multiple myeloma: a prospective comparative trial. Abst Blood, 96: 583a, 2000.
66. Szczepek AJ, Belch AR, Pilarski LM. Expression of IL-6 and IL-6 Receptors by Circulating Clonotypic B Cells in Multiple Myeloma: Potential for Autocrine and Paracrine Networks. Exp Hematol, 29: 1076-1081, 2001.
67. Turley EA, Belch AR, Poppema S, Pilarski LM. Expression and function of a receptor for hyaluronan-mediated motility (RHAMM) on normal and malignant B lymphocytes. Blood, 81: 446-453, 1993.
68. Bataille R, Chappard D, Marcelli C, Dessauw P, Baldet P, Sany J, Alexandre C. Recruitment of new osteoblasts and osteoclasts is the earliest critical event in the pathogenesis of human multiple myeloma. J Clin Invest, 88: 62-66, 1991.
69. Rondelli D, Bandini G, Cavo M, Re F, Motta MR, Senese B, Leopardi G, Stanzini M, Tura S. Discrepancy between serological complete remission and concomitant new bone lytic lesions after infusion of escalating low doses of donor lymphocytres in multiple myeloma: a case report. Bone Marrow Transp, 24: 685-687, 1999.
70. Borrello MA, Phipps RP. The B/macrophage cell: an elusive link between CD5+ B lymphocytes and macrophages. Immunol Today, 17: 471-475, 1996.
71. Eilion G, Mundy GR. Direct resorption of bone by human breast cancer cells in vitro. Nature, 276: 726-728, 1978.
72. Sanchez-Sweatman OH, Orr FW, Singh G. Human metastatic prostate PC3 cell lines degrade bone using matrix metalloproteinases. Invasion Metastasis 18: 297-305, 1998.
73. Sanchez-Sweatman OH, Singh G, Kruger A, Khoka R, Orr FW. Human skeletal metastatic cell lines directly degrade bone matrix using matrix metalloproteinases. Invasion Metastasis, 18: 297-305, 1999.
74. Rothschild BM, Hershkovitz I, Dutour O. Clues potentially distinguishing lytic lesions of multiple myeloma from those of metastatic carcinoma. Am J Phys Anthropo 106: 241-250, 1998.
75. Bataille R, Chappard D, Alexandre C, Dessauw P, Sany J. Importance of quantitative histology of bone changes in monoclonal gammopathy. Br J Cancer 53: 805-810, 1986.
76. Thiele J, Arenz B, Klein H, Vierbuchen M, Zankovich R, Fischer R. Differentiation of plasma cell infiltrates in the bone marrow: A clinicopathological study on 80 patients including immunohistochemistry and morphology. Virchows Archiv A Pathol Anat Histopathol, 412: 553-562, 1988.
77. Roux C, Ravaud P, Cohen-Solal M, de Vernejoul MC, Guillemant S, Cherruau B, Delmas P, Dougados M, Amor B. Biologic, histologic and densitometric effecs of oral risedronate on bone in patients with multiple myeloma. Bone, 15: 41-49, 1994.

78. Bartl R, Frisch B, Diem H, Mundel M, Fateh-Moghadam A. Bone marrow histology and serum beta 2 microglobulin in multiple myeloma - a new prognostic strategy. Eur J Haematol, 43: 88-98, 1989.
79. Valentin-Opran A, Charhon SA, Meunier PJ, Edouard CM, Arlot ME. Quantitative histology of myeloma-induced bone changes. Br J Haematol, 52: 601-610, 1982.
80. Dhodapkar MV, Weinstein RS, Tricot G, Jagannath S, Parfitt AM, Manolagas SC, Barlogie B. Biologic and therapeutic determinants of bone mineral density in multiple myeloma. Leuk Lymphoma, 32: 121-127. 1998.
81. Diamond T, Levy S, Day P, Barbagallo S, Manoharan A, Kwan YK. Biochemical, histomorphometric and densitometric changes in patients with multiple myeloma: effects of glucocorticosteroid therapy and disease activity. Br J Haematol, 97: 641-648, 1997.
82. Mariette X, Bergot C, Ravaud P, Roux C, Laval-Jeantet M, Brouet JC, Fermand JP. Evolution of bone densitometry in patients with myeloma treated with conventional or intensive chemotherapy. Cancer, 76: 1559-1563, 1995.
83. Rossi JF, Bataille R, Chappard D, Alexandre C, Janbon C. B cell malignancies presenting with unusual bone involvement and mimicking multiple myeloma. Am J Med, 83: 10-16, 1987.
84. Aghai E, Avni G, Lurie M, Quitt M, Hornstein L, Froom P. Bone marrow biopsy in multiple myeloma: a clinical pathological study. Israel J.Med Sci, 24: 298-301, 1988.
85. Mariette X, Khalifa P, Ravaud P, Frija J, Laval-Jeantet M, Chastang C, Brouet JC, and Fermand JP. Bone densitometry in patients with multiple myeloma. Am J.Med, 93: 595-598, 1992.
86. Barlogie B. High-dose therapy and innovative approaches to treatment of multiple myeloma. Semin Hematol, 38: 21-27, 2001.
87. Smith DB, Scarffe JH, Eddleston B. The prognostic significance of x-ray changes at presentation and reassessment in patients with multiple myeloma. Hematol Oncol, 6: 1-6, 1988.
88. Wulfeck DW, Williams TE. Paradoxical poor prognosis of myeloma patients who demonstrate complete healing of bone lesions following treatment. Ky Med Assoc, 92: 136-139, 1994.
89. Sebes JI, Niell HB, Palmieri GM, Reidy TJ. Skeletal surveys in multiple myeloma. Radiologic-clinical correlation. Skeletal Radiol, 15: 354-359, 1986.
90. Rosen LS, Gordon D, Kaminski M, Howell A, Belch A, Mackey JA, Apffelsteadt J, Coleman RE, Reitsma DJ, Chen BL, Ambros Y. Zoledronic acid versus pamidronate in the treatment of skeletal metastases in patients with breast cancer or osteolytic lesions of multiple myeloma: a phase III, double-blind, comparative trial. Cancer J, 7: 377-387, 2001.
91. Raje N, Anderson KC. Introduction: the evolving role of bisphosphonate therapy in multiple myeloma. Blood, 96: 381-383. 2000.
92. Tricot G. New insights into role of microenvironment in multiple myeloma. Lancet, 355: 248-250. 2000.
93. Karadag A, Scutt AM, Croucher PI. Human myeloma cells promote the recruitment of osteoblast precursors: mediation by interleukin-6 and soluble interleukin-6 receptor. J Bone Mineral Res, 15: 1935-1943, 2000.
94. Michigami T, Shimizu N, Williams PJ, Niewolna M, Dallas SL, Mundy GR, Yoneda T. Cell-cell contact between marrow stromal cells and myeloma cells via VCAM-1 and alpha (4) beta (1) integrin enhances production of osteoclast-stimulating activity. Blood, 96: 1953-1960, 2000.

95. Derenne S, Amiot M, Barille S, Collette M, Robillard N, Berthaud P, Harousseau JL, Bataille R. Zoledronate is a potent inhibitor of myeloma cell growth and secretion of IL-6 and MMP-1 by the tumoral environment. J Bone Min Res, 14: 2048-2056, 1999.
96. Berenson JR, Lichtenstein A, Porter L, Dimopoulos MA, Bordoni R, GeorgeS, Lipton A, Keller A, Ballester O, Kovacs MJ, et al. Efficacy of pamidronate in reducing skeletal events in patients with advanced multiple myeloma. Myeloma Aredia Study Group. N Engl J Med, 334: 488-493. 1996.
97. Adam Z, Prokes B, Hajek D, Vorlicek J. Increasing bone density in myeloma patients after the administration of clodronate. Acta Med Austriaca, 22: 9-12, 1995.
98. Popovic SV, Coulterjohn N, Lhotak S, Duivenvoorden WC, Orr FW, Singh G. Morphological, histomorphometric and microstructural alterations in human bone metastasisfrom breast carcinoma. Bone, 31: 529-535, 2002.
99. McDonnell GD, Dunstan CR, Evans RA, Carter JN, Hills E, Wong SY, McNeil DR. Quantitative bone histology in the hypercalcemia of malignant disease. J Clin Endocrinol Metab, 55: 1066-1072, 1982.
100. Sailer M, Vykoupil KF, Peest D, Coldeway R, Deicher H, Georgii A. Prognostic relevance of a histologic classification system applied in bone marrow biopsies from patients with multiple myeloma: a histopathological evaluation of biopsies from 153 untreated patients. Eur J Haematol, 54: 137-146, 1995.
101. Mundy GR, Raisz LG, Cooper RA, Schecter GP, Salmon SE. Evidence for the secretion of an osteoclast stimulating factor in myeloma. N Engl J Med, 291: 1041-1046, 1974.
102. Kyle RA, Greipp PR. Smoldering multiple myeloma. New Eng J Med, 302: 1347-1349, 1980.
103. Kyle RA. Monoclonal gammopathy of undetermined significance. Natural history in 241 cases. Am J Med, 64: 814-826, 1978.
104. Bataille R, Chappard D, Basle MF. Quantifiable excess of bone resorption in monoclonal gammopathy is an early symptom of malignancy: a prospective study of 87 bone biopsies. Blood, 87: 4762-4769, 1996.
105. Frassanito MA, Cusmai A, Iodice G, Dammaco F. Autocrine interleukin-6 production and highly malignant multiple myeloma: relation with resistance to drug-induced apoptosis. Blood, 97: 483-489, 2001.
106. Barille S, Bataille R, Amiot M. The role of interleukin-6 and interleukin-6/interleukin-6 receptor α complex in the pathogenesis of multiple myeloma. Eur Cytokine Netw, 11: 546-551, 2000.
107. Thabard W, Barille S, Collette M, Harousseau JL, Rapp MJ, Bataille R, Amiot M. Myeloma cells release soluble interleukin-6 Ralpha in relation to disease progression by two distinct mechanisms: alternative splicing and proteolytic cleavage. Clin Cancer Res, 5: 2693-2697, 1999.
108. Iwasaki T, Hamano T, Ogata A, Kakishita E. Clinical significance of interleukin-6 gene expression in the bone marrow of patients with multiple myeloma. Int J Hematol, 70: 16-38, 2001.
109. Anderson KC, Lust JA. Role of cytokines in multiple myeloma. Semin Hematol, 36: 14-20, 1999.
110. Xu FH, Sharma S, Gardner A, Tu V, Raitano A, Sawyers C, and Lichtenstein A. Interleukin-6-induced inhibition of multiple myeloma cell apoptosis: support for the hypothesis that protection is mediated via inhibition of the JNK/SAPK pathway. Blood, 92: 241-251, 1998.
111. Sati HI, Apperley JF, Greaves M, Lawry J, Gooding R, Russell RG, Croucher PI. Interleukin-6 is expressed by plasma cells from patients with multiple myeloma and

monoclonal gammopathy of undetermined significance. Br J Haematol, 101: 287-295, 1998.
112. Treon SP, Anderson KC. Interleukin-6 in multiple myeloma and related plasma cell dyscrasias. Curr Opin Hematol. 5: 42-48, 1998.
113. Hata H, Xiao H, Petrucci MT, Woodliff J, Chang R, and Epstein J. Interleukin-6 gene expression in multiple myeloma: a characteristic of immature tumor cells. Blood, 81: 3357-3364, 1993.
114. Roodman GD. Cell biology of the osteoclast. Exp Hematol, 27: 1229-1241, 1996.
115. Dankbar B, Padro T, Leo R, Feldmann B, Kropff M, Mesters RM, Serve H, Berdel WE, Kienast J. Vascular endothelial growth factor and interleukin-6 in paracrine tumor - stromal cell interactions in multiple myeloma. Blood, 95: 2630-2636, 2000.
116. Selby P, Zulian G, Forgeson G, Nandi A, Milan S, Meldrum M, Viner C, Osborne R, Malpas JS, McElwain TJ. The development of high dose melphalan and of autologous bone marrow transplantation in the treatment of multiple myeloma: Royal Marsden and St Bartholomew's Hospital studies. Hematol Oncol, 6: 173-179, 1998.
117. Yaccoby S, Barlogie B, Epstein J. Depletion of myeloma plasma cells prevents in vivo development of myeloma. Abst Proc Am Assoc Cancer Res, 39: 589, 1998.
118. Yaccoby S, Barlogie B, Epstein J. Primary myeloma cells growing in SCID-Hhu mice: A model for studying the biology and treatment of myeloma and its manifestations. Blood, 92: 2908-2913, 1998.
119. Pilarski LM, Gillitzer R, Zola H, Shortman K, Scollay R. Selective expression of CD45 (T200) antigens during human thymocyte differentiation. Eur J Immunol, 19: 589-597, 1988.
120. Scollay R, Smith J, Stauffer V. Dynamics of early T cells: prothymocyte migration and proliferation in the adult mouse thymus. Immunol Rev, 91: 129-157, 1986.
121. Scollay R, Wilson A, D'Amico A, Kelly K, Egerton M, Pearse M, Wu L, Shortman K. Developmental status and reconstitution potential of subpopulations of murine thymocytes. Immunol Rev, 104: 81-120, 2001.
122. Deenick EK, Hasbold J, and Hodgkin PD. Switching to igG3, IgG2b and IgA is division linked and independent, revealing a stochastic framework for describing differentiation. J Immunol, 163: 4707-4714, 1999.
123. Vaananen HK, Zhao H, Mulari M, Halleen JM. The cell biology of osteoclast function. J Cell Sci, 113: 377-381, 2000.
124. Hofbauer LC, Khosla S, Dunstan CR, Lacey DL, Boyle WJ, Riggs L. The roles of osteoprotegerin and osteoprotegerin ligand in the paracrine regulation of bone resorption. J Bone Min Res, 15: 2-12, 2000.
125. Li J, Sarosi I, Yan XQ, Morony S, Capparelli C, Tan HL, McCabe S, Elliott R, Scully S, Van G, et al. RANK is the intrinsic hematopoietic cell surface receptor that controls osteoclastogenesis and regulation of bone mass and calcium metabolism. Proc Nat Acad Sci USA 97: 1566-1571, 2000.
126. Shaloub V, Faust J, Boyle WJ, Dustan CR, Kelley M, Kaufman S, Scully S, Van G, Lacey DL. Osteoprotegerin and osteoprotegerin ligand effects on osteoclast formation from human peripheral blood mononuclear cell precursors. J Cell Biochem, 72: 251-261, 1999.
127. Croucher PI, Shipman C, Lippett J, Perry M, Kewal A, Hijzen A, van Beek EJR, Holen I, Skerry TM, Dunstan CR, Russell GR, van Camp B, Vanderkerken K. Osteoprotegerin inhibits the development of osteolytic bone disease in multiple myeloma. Blood, 98: 3534-3540, 2001.

128. Manaabe N, Kawaguchi H, Chikuda H, Miyaura C, Inada M, Nagai R, Nabeshima YI, Nakamura K, Sinclair A, Schuermann RH, Kuro-o M. Connection between B lymphocyte and osteoclast differentiation pathways. J Immunol, 167: 2625-2631, 2001
129. Sezer O, Heider U, Jakob C, Zavarski I, Possinger K, Sers C, Krenn V. Immunocytochemistry reveals RANKL expression of myeloma cells. Blood, 99: 4646-4647, 2002.
130. Sezer O, Heider U, Zavarski I, Kuhne CA, Hofbauer LC. RANK ligand and osteoprotegerin in myeloma bone disease. Blood, 101: 2094-2098, 2003.
131. Seidel C. Hjertner O, Abildgaard N, Heickendorff L, Westin J, Nielson JL, Hjorth-Hansen H, Waage A, Sundan A, Borset M, Nordic Study Group. Serum osteoprotegerin levels are reduced in patients with multiple myeloma and lytic bone disease. Blood, 98: 2269-2271, 2001.
132. Sandal T, Seidel C, Hjertner O, Plesner T, Sanderson RD, Waage A, Borset M, Sundan A. Osteoprotegerin is bound, internalized, and degraded by multiple myeloma cells. Blood, 100: 3002-3007, 2002.
133. Lipton A, Ali M, Leitzel K, Chinchilli V, Witters L, Engle L, Holloway D, Bekker P, Dunstan CR. Serum osteoprotegerin levels in healthy controls and cancer patients. Clin Cancer Rese 8: 2306-2310, 2002.
134. Faust J, Hunt P, Scully S, Shaloub V. Multiple myeloma cells and cells of the human osteoclast lineage share morphological and cell surface markers. J Cell Biochem, 71: 559-568, 1998.
135. Gregoretti MG, Bergui L, Aragno M, Cremona O, Marchisio PC, Caligaris-Cappio F. Osteoclast precursors circulate in the peripheral blood of patients with aggressive multiple myeloma. Leukemia, 9: 1392-1397, 1995.
136. Ely SA, Knowles DM. Expression of CD56/neural cell adhesion molecule correlates with the presence of lytic bone lesions in multiple myeloma and distinguishes myeloma from monoclonal gammopathy of undetermined significance and lymphomas with plasmacytoid differentiation. Am J Pathol, 160: 1293-1299, 2002.

Chapter 8

ANGIOGENESIS AND LYMPHANGIOGENESIS IN METASTATIC BONE DISEASE: A MATTER OF NETWORKING

Gabri Van Der Pluijm and Jeroen Buijs
Leiden University Medical Cente,rDepartment of Endocrinology C4-R86, Leiden, The Netherlands
Leiden University Medical Center,Department of Endocrinology C4-R, Leiden, The Netherlands

1. INTRODUCTION

In healthy adults, (lymph)angiogenesis is limited to processes of repair (wound healing) and is restricted to the female reproductive tract (ovulatory cycle). In normal tissues, vascular quiescence is maintained by the dominant influence of endogenous angiogenesis inhibitors over angiogenic stimuli. In pathologic conditions, however, this delicate balance can be disrupted and lead to initiation and stimulation of blood or lymphatic vessel formation ('angiogenic switch'). Neovascularization or angiogenesis -the formation of new blood vessels from pre-existing ones- is vital for the growth of tumors, providing a lifeline for sustenance and waste disposal. It is, therefore, tempting to speculate that interactions between osteotropic cancer cells and the (a)cellular bone marrow stoma lead to differential expression of (lymph)angiogenic factors and their inhibitors in the bone microenvironment, thus explaining -at least in part- the observed bone tropism by a limited number of carcinomas.

Osteotropic cancers can generate a microcirculation comparable to processes involved to the development of a vascular system during embryogenesis. In this chapter, we will discuss the role of angiogenesis, lymphangiogenesis, postnatal vasculogenesis and vasculogenic mimicry in

G. Singh and W. Orr (eds.), Bone Metastasis and Molecular Mechanisms, 139-162.

Angiogenesis or neovascularization, the formation of blood capillaries from pre-existing blood vessels, extends and remodels the primitive vasculature giving rise to a complex vascular network (Figure 1). Angiogenesis is a multi-step process that is regulated by soluble factors as well as by cell-matrix interactions (8, 12, 13, 17-20). Activation of endothelial cells by angiogenic stimuli derived from non-endothelial cells results in expression of proteolytic enzymes and site-directed proteolytic activity. After degradation of the basement membrane, endothelial cells adhere to the surrounding matrix, migrate towards angiogenic stimuli and invade the surrounding tissue. Proliferation of endothelial cells in the sprouting capillary results in extension and elongation of the sprout and eventually a lumen is formed. Several sprouts will join to form a loop in which blood can circulate, resulting in vascularization of the tissue. Finally, pericytes are recruited to stabilize the newly formed vessels. Angiopoietins 1 and 2, PDGF, and members of the transforming growth factor-β (TGF-β) superfamily are crucial to this final step of angiogenesis. Angiopoietin 1 and PDGF are involved in the reciprocal communication between endothelial cells and pericytes. In contrast, angiopoietin 2 acts both as an inhibitor and stimulator of angiogenesis, while, in the presence of VEGF-A, angiopoietin 2 stimulates detachment of peri-endothelial cells, thereby promoting angiogenesis.

In addition to blood vessels, lymphatic vessels belong to the vascular circulatory system. Although the lymphatic vessels were discovered in the early 17th century, relatively little is known about their formation, maintenance, and their exact role in disease (8, 12, 18, 20, 21). This is mainly due to the lack of specific markers. Only recently have researchers identified molecules whose expression is restricted to the lymphatic endothelium. It has been proposed that isolated lymph sacs originate by endothelial budding from embryonic veins (8, 12, 18, 20, 21 22). The peripheral lymphatic system spreads from primary lymph sacs by endothelial sprouting into the surrounding tissues or organs. Alternatively, it has also been suggested that lymph sacs arise from the mesenchyme from precursor cells (lymphangioblasts) independent of the veins but that they form venous connections later. Although lymphatic vessels share several properties with blood vessels (e.g. lining by endothelium), there are clear differences. Blood vessels have a continuous or fenestrated basement membrane and tight interendothelial junctions, which make the vessel wall selectively permeable to cells, fluids, and molecules, whereas lymphatic vessels constitute a relative barrier for interstitial fluid (8, 12, 18, 20, 21). In addition, lymphatic vessels have complex overlapping intercellular junctions and specialized anchoring filaments which hold the vessel open as tissue pressure rises. Liquids, macromolecules, and migrating cells pass through the blood capillary endothelia, enter the tissues, and are gradually absorbed into the lymphatic system. The fluid is transported via the lymphatic capillaries into the collecting vessels and through the lymph nodes eventually returning to the circulation (8). The blood vascular endothelium is a relatively leak-proof, nonthrombogenic surface, with tightly regulated flow and intraluminal pressure, whereas the lymphatics, in contrast, are a low-flow, low-pressure system in close contact with the extracellular matrix (8, 12, 18, 20, 21).

3. ANGIOGENESIS IN TUMOR GROWTH AND METASTASIS.

Tumor blood and lymphatic vessels can grow by sprouting, intussusception or by incorporating bone marrow-derived endothelial precursor cells into growing vessels (postnatal vasculogenesis, *de novo* formation of blood vessels by hemangioblasts) (8, 18, 20, 22). Angiogenesis is essential for tumor growth and metastasis. Angiogenesis is a complex, multistep process that involves dissolution of the basement membrane of the vessel and extracellular matrix degradation, migration and proliferation of endothelial cells, capillary differentiation, stabilization and anastomosis.

Inducers and inhibitors of endothelial proliferation, migration and differentiation tightly regulate these processes. In the adult, the vascular network is relatively stable and vascular turnover is extremely low and is considered to be nearly quiescent. With the exception of the female reproductive cycle, angiogenesis in adults occurs only under pathological conditions such as wound healing and tumor growth, when the balance is shifted in favor of angiogenesis either by increased levels of angiogenic inducers or decreased levels of angiogenic inhibitors. In malignancy, tumor cells can switch from an angiogenesis-inhibiting phenotype to an angiogenesis-stimulating phenotype, a process which is referred to as the *angiogenic switch* (23-25).

Angiogenesis is essential for tumor growth as it provides oxygenation and nourishment of the tumor and allows removal of waste products. Angiogenesis thus allows the tumor cells to express their critical growth advantage and also permits the establishment of continuity with the existing vasculature of the host. In addition, increased angiogenesis coincides with increased tumor cell entry into the circulation and thereby facilitates metastasis. A strong correlation has been found between the density of microvessels in primary breast and prostate tumors and nodal metastases and patient survival, as in other malignancies (17, 26-49).

Tumors produce and secrete a variety of pro-angiogenic molecules, incuding members of the VEGF family (Figure 2). VEGF-A is a specific endothelial cell mitogen and inducer of angiogenesis. It also potently induces vascular permeability to macromolecules and is, therefore, also known as vascular permeability factor (VPF). VEGF-B binds to VEGFR-1 whereas VEGF-C binds to VEGFR-3 (flt-4).The latter receptor is specific for lymphatic endothelium and VEGF-C stimulates the growth of lymphatic vessels. VEGF-D is closely related to VEGF-C and bind to the same receptor. Proteolytically processed VEGF-C and D are also able to bind to VEGFR-2 but have lower affinity and are, therefore, weakly angiogenic (6) (Figure 2).

In addition, it is becoming increasingly clear that various malignant tumors can acquire a microcirculation by recruiting circulating endothelial progenitor cells or hemangioblasts from peripheral blood (Figure 1). Xenotransplant models have convincingly demonstrated that postnatal vascularization in various cancers does not rely exclusively on sprouting from pre-existing blood or lymphatic vessels. Instead, endothelial progenitors circulate from the bone marrow to incorporate into and thus contribute to postnatal physiological and pathological neovascularization, which is consistent with postnatal vasculogenesis (2-4, 6, 9, 50-52). Tumors are, therefore, capable of stimulating *de novo* formation of blood capillaries that can subsequently fuse with the existing vasculature, thus connecting the tumor to the vasculature of the body.

4. THE EMERGING ROLE OF LYMPHANGIOGENESIS AND TUMOR METASTASIS

Metastasis of osteotropic cancers, like breast and prostate carcinoma, occurs in part through the lymphatic system, and the extent of lymph node involvement is a key prognostic factor for the disease. While the importance and prognostic significance of the ability of tumor cells to stimulate angiogenesis has been firmly established, the significance of lymphangiogenesis has not been well documented. This has been mainly due to the lack of consistent data with reliable lymphatic endothelial cell markers. However, the recent discovery of novel lymphatic endothelial cell markers (e.g. prox-1, LYVE-1, VEGFR3 and podoplanin) have led to the demonstration of newly formed lymphatic vessels within the bulk of the tumor in animal models and human neoplasms, and the characterization of the VEGF-C/VEGFR-3 pathway (20, 53-57).

In vivo studies have shown that the soluble protein growth factors, VEGF-C and VEGF-D, and their cognate receptor tyrosine kinase, VEGF receptor-3 (VEGFR-3), are critical regulators of lymphangiogenesis. Like VEGF-A, VEGF-C stimulates the migration of endothelial cells and increases vascular permeability and endothelial cell proliferation but at higher concentrations than VEGF (8, 10, 18). These signals for endothelial cells are probably mediated through VEGFR-2 in blood vascular endothelial cells, and generally via VEGFR-3 in the lymphatic endothelial cells (8, 10, 18, 58-61). Unlike VEGF, the expression of VEGF-C is not regulated by hypoxia (61). The angiogenic versus lymphangiogenic responses to VEGF-C may depend on the degree of proteolytic processing of its precursor and on the expression of its receptors in the blood versus lymphatic endothelial cells of the target tissue (8, 10, 12, 18, 19). VEGF-C also has synergistic effects with VEGF, during the induction of angiogenesis, and this effect is more prominent in cells expressing both of its receptors (12, 19). In addition, VEGF-C can compete with VEGF in binding to VEGFR-2.

VEGF-D (also known as c-*fos*-induced growth factor or FIGF) (1, 62, 63) shares 61% sequence identity with VEGF-C, and these two growth factors bind to the same receptors on human endothelial cells. VEGF-D has been shown to be able to stimulate the proliferation of endothelial cells, and it shows angiogenic properties *in vitro* and *in vivo* (11). Like VEGF-C, it was also shown to be lymphangiogenic when overexpressed in skin keratinocytes (10).

Skobe and co-workers (56) demonstrated the presence of lymphangiogenesis within the peripheral areas of MDA-MB-435/GFP tumors, suggesting the production of lymphangiogenic factors in this metastatic tumor. Overexpression of VEGF-C resulted in enlargement of peritumoral lymphatic vessels and in increased intratumoral lymphangiogenesis –identifying VEGF-C as a potent tumor lymphangiogenesis factor.

Tumor-associated lymphatic vessels contribute to the efficient transport of fluids and macromolecules and are, therefore, of great importance for overall tumor physiology and drug delivery, but it may not be critical for tumor dissemination (56). Nevertheless, the formation of an intratumoral lymphatic network, whether functional in fluid transport or not, might promote metastatic tumor spread by creating increased opportunities for metastatic tumor cells to leave the primary tumor site.

Skobe and coworkers (56) demonstrated that the increased density of lymphatic vessels within VEGF-C–overexpressing breast cancers was associated with a significantly increased incidence of metastases in regional lymph nodes. Therefore, these findings provide a novel mechanistic insight into the reported correlation of VEGF-C expression in the primary tumors with high incidence of lymph node metastases in, for instance, breast and prostate carcinoma (64). Moreover, a recent study found that VEGF-C expression was only detectable in node-positive breast cancers, whereas expression of VEGF was detected in both node-positive and node-negative tumors. VEGF-C may promote the incidence of lymphatic metastases, thereby facilitating tumor cell entry into the lymphatics.

In addition to these studies, Kinoshita and co-workers found that VEGF-C may not be directly involved in vascular spread but may act as promising marker to predict recurrence, thus implying that VEGF-C can also play a role in metastatic growth (55).

5. VASCULAR NETWORKS IN OSTEOTROPIC CANCERS AND EXPERIMENTALLY-INDUCED BONE METASTASES.

The dissemination of cancer cells can occur directly into the local tissue, via blood vessels (hematogeneous spread) and lymphatics (lymphatic spread), or by invasion of body cavities (18). Tumor-induced angiogenesis and the expression of various angiogenic factors like VEGF-A, bFGF and their receptors have been identified as prognostic indicators of poor prognosis and disease recurrence.

The lymphangiogenic concept described above is supported by our observations that thin meshworks exist in experimentally-induced bone metastases from MDA-MB-231 cells (Figure 3) (65, 66) and in primary breast carcinomas and their lymph node metastases in patients (Figure 4, upper panels). Experimentally-induced bone metastases from human breast (MDA-MB-231) and prostate cancer (PC-3M-Pro4) in nude mice strongly stimulate angiogenesis (CD31+ blood vessels, Figure 3c) and induce the formation of complex three-dimensional networks (Figure 3d) (65, 66). In these animals, MDA-MB-231 breast cancer cells in mestastatic lesions express a variety of pro-angiogenic factors, including VEGF-A, -B and –C. Strikingly, we found that the expression of VEGF-A, VEGF-B and VEGF-C is strongly and significantly (VEGF-A, -B) upregulated in bone metastases when compared with soft tissue metastases, suggesting that tumor-bone (marrow) interactions play a decisive role in colonization and/or subsequent invasive growth of osteotropic cancers (66). In primary tumors and lymph node metastases in breast cancer patients various Periodic Acid Schiff positive (PAS+) patterns, including PAS+ meshworks, are frequently observed. These PAS+ patterns are often characterized by the lack of Flt-4/VEGFR3 expression, patchy expression of PECAM-1/CD 31 and vimentin, and the continuous expression of Smooth Muscle Actin (SMA).

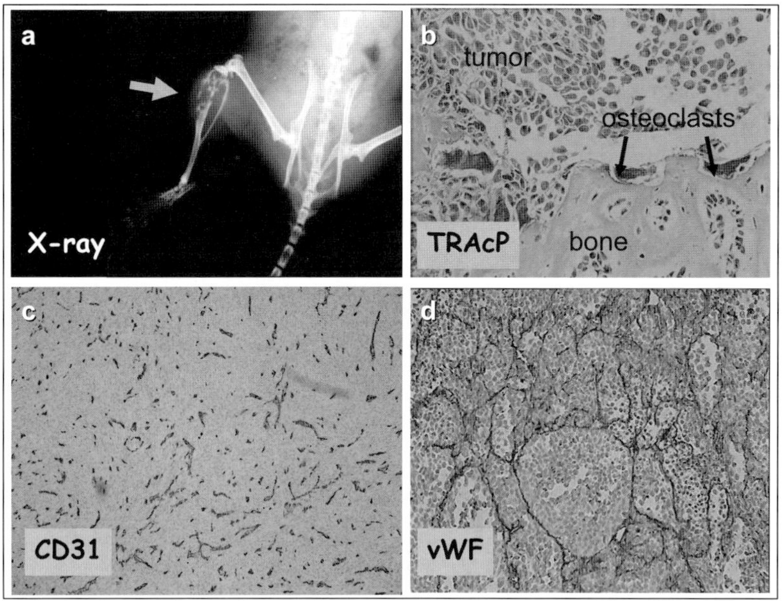

Figure 3. Osteolytic bone metastasis in the tibia of a nude mouse after intracardiac inoculation of 100,000 human MDA-MB-231 breast cancer cells. A. Radiograph showing multiple osteolytic lesion in bone, B. MDA-MB-231 cells have almost completely replaced the bone marrow and strongly induce the formation of Tartrate-Resistant Acid Phosphatase (TRAcP) osteoclasts that resorb surrounding bone, C. Tumor blood caplillaries in a bone lesion stained by the CD31 or PECAM-1 antibody MP-12, D. A section of a bone metastasis stained for von Willebrand factor (vWF) showing a network of interconnected loops.

We have recently found that the prognosis of the patient is inversely correlated with the complexity of the PAS+ meshwork in lymph node metastases (Figure 4, lower panels. Buijs et al., submitted for publication). Furthermore, the presence of a PAS+ network, the most complex PAS+ pattern, in either primary tumor or lymph node metastases from invasive ductal carcinoma of the breast, is one of the three independent factors associated with the recurrence of a distant metastasis and survival (Buijs et al., submitted for publication). The presence of lumina in the PAS+ meshwork might be indicative for septa that could facilitate perfusion and dissemination of cancer cells. Indeed, tumor cells were frequently present in the lumina, whereas, erythrocytes were occasionally found in these structures. In addition, Foss and co-workers provided evidence that PAS+ extracellular septa can be particularly favorable substrates for the in-growth of angiogenic, and possibly lymphatic, vessels (67). Consequently, tumors that contain these PAS+ structures might be more aggressive, as these structures provide better means for (blood) vessel in-growth than tumors lacking these structures. Alternatively, it cannot be excluded that highly malignant breast cancer cells can acquire an invasive, mesenchymal phenotype, a process called epithelium-to-mesenchyme transition (EMT). It is, therefore, tempting to speculate that tumor cells that aligne hollow tubular structures are phenotypically distinct from other tumor cells. The generation of such a PAS+ network by genetically deregulated, aggressive tumor cells was termed 'vasculogenic mimicry' to emphasize their *de novo* generation without participation of endothelial cells and independent of angiogenesis (68-70). Recent reports suggest that vasculogenic mimicry also exists in ovarian (71), prostate and breast cancer (1, 70, 72-74). After establishing an inflammatory breast cancer (IBC) xenograft with vasculogenic mimicry features, Shirakawa and co-workers examined surgically resected breast cancers and classified 7.9 % as exhibiting vasculogenic mimicry (73). The existence of vasculogenic mimicry increased the likelihood of hematogenous spread and gave a poorer prognosis for the patient.

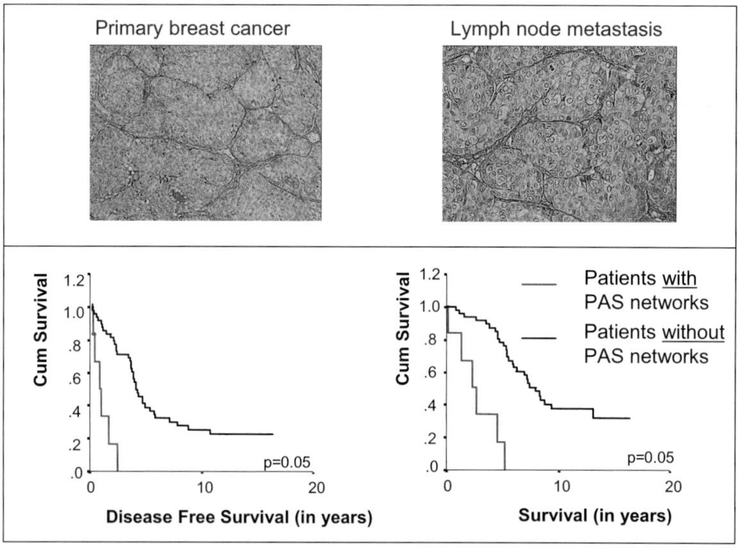

Figure 4. The presence of a periodic acid Schiff (PAS)+ network in the primary tumor or lymph node metastases from invasive ductal carcinoma of the breast (upper panels) is one of the independent factors associated with the recurrence of a distant metastasis and survival (lower panels) as determined by Cumulative disease free survival and overall survival (Buijs et al., submitted for publication).

The lack of continuous Flt4/VEGFR3 expression (VEGF-C receptor and lymphatic marker) in the PAS+ network may indicate that these structures are complex and do not only represent the lymphatic vasculature. If the septa consist of two layers of ECM elaborated by opposing layers of tumor cell, the layers could separate from another, forming channels and laminar openings. Such openings could particularly lead to capillary growth. The patchy expression of the endothelial marker, CD31/PECAM-1, is in agreement with this hypothesis.

The presence of PAS+ networks, in either primary tumor or lymph node metastases from invasive ductal carcinoma of the breast, is one of the three independent factors associated with the recurrence of a distant metastasis. Moreover, the presence of a PAS+ network in a positive lymph node is the factor most strongly associated with recurrence.

6. OPTICAL IMAGING, A NOVEL NON-INVASIVE TECHNIQUE FOR MONITORING BONE METASTASIS; EVIDENCE FOR AN ANGIOGENIC SWITCH.

Investigation of the pathogenesis of bone metastasis, the involvement of specific genes (functional genomics) and evaluation of therapeutic agents would greatly benefit from a method that could non-invasively image cancer cells *in vivo*. Furthermore, the development of novel anti-cancer and anti-angiogenic strategies requires more sensitive and less invasive methods to detect and monitor *in vivo* minimal residual disease in (breast) cancer metastasis.

Injection of cancer cell lines into the left cardiac ventricle of immunodeficient (*nu/nu*) mice is a widely used animal model of bone/bone marrow metastasis (65, 66, 75-79). This experimental setting closely resembles the clinical situation of minimal residual disease after removal of the primary tumor. However, detection of bone metastasis by radiography does not make it an ideal model of minimal residual disease.

In fact, radiologically evident bone metastases are a late and macroscopic event in the evolution of metastatic bone disease. Thus, the model lacks the sensitivity that would be necessary to dissect the initial processes, such as the *angiogenic switch*, essential for tumor progression. Furthermore, the radiological detection and measurement of skeletal metastases do not represent actual tumor burden. As a result the size of the bone lesions are not only dependent on tumor cell numbers, but also on the ability of the cancer cells to excrete factors that stimulate bone remodeling during the course of the experiment. Only a parallel histomorphometric analysis allows the distinction between a therapeutic effect exerted directly on tumor cells or indirectly through inhibition of bone resorption.

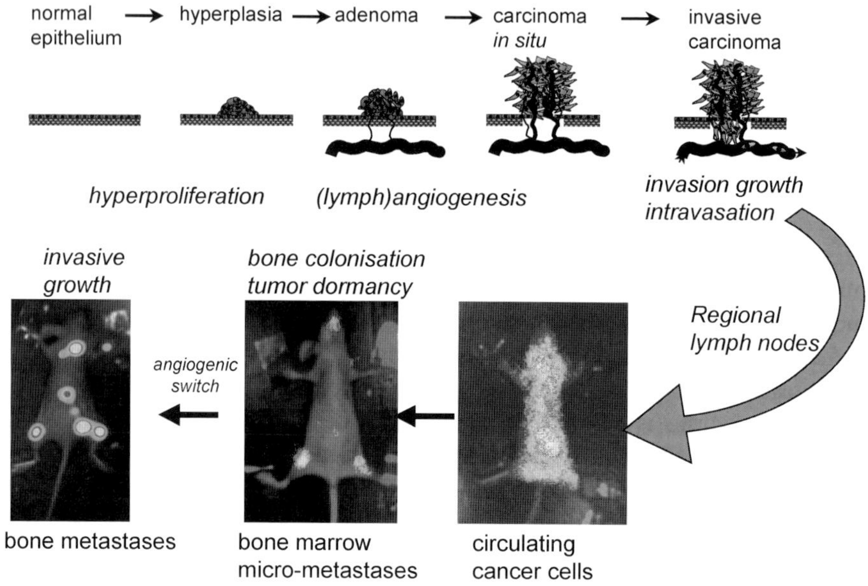

Figure 7. Sequential steps involved in carcinogenesis, dissemination, and metastasis. Carcinomas develop from normal epithelium and undergo sequential genetic changes that, in interaction with the (a) cellular microenvironment, can lead to dissemination and (bone) metastases. The ability of cancer cells to stimulate angiogenesis and lymphangiogenesis at the primary and metastastic sites is of key interest for successful growth and metastasis. Particularly, members of the TGF-β superfamily are involved during carcinogenesis at the primary site and in the devlopment of bone metastasis. Perturbation of TGF-βsignalling cascades in osteotropic cancers may sensitize these tumor cells to growth signals that are intrinsic (or characteristic) to the bone/bone marrow microenvironment, leading to accelerated, invasive growth.

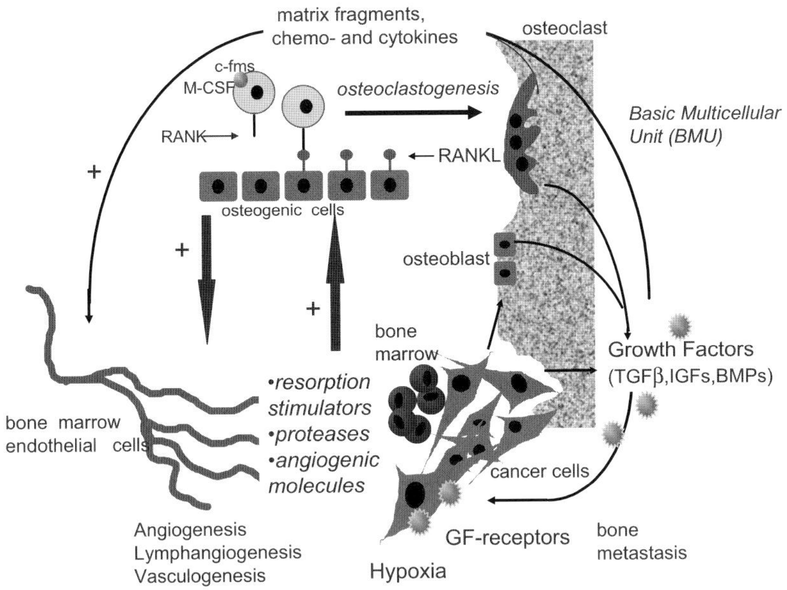

Figure 8. Schematic overview of the vicious cycle of bone metastasis and invasive growth by (breast) cancer cells in bone marrow. Interactions between cancer cells and the bone/bone marrow mivcroenvironment are prerequisites for skeletal metastasis. Soluble factors, including matrix components that are released from the bone surface or produced by supportive bone marrow cells (e.g. TGF-β, IGFs, BMPs) as well as tumor cell - stromal cell interactions are prerequisites for successful colonization and subsequent invasive growth of osteotropic cancers. Acquisition of a microcirculation by angiogenesis, lymphangiogenesis, vasculogenesis and/or vasculogenic mimicry is crucial for the metastatic growth of cancer cells.

REFERENCES

1. Achen M, Stacker GSA. The vascular endothelial growth factor family; proteins which guide the development of the vasculature. Int J Exp Pathol, 79: 255-265, 1998.
2. Asahara T, Masuda H, Takahashi T, Kalka C, Pastore C, Silver M, Kearne M, Magner M, Isner JM. Bone marrow origin of endothelial progenitor cells responsible for postnatal vasculogenesis in physiological and pathological neovascularization. Circ Res, 85: 221-228, 1999.
3. Bertolini F, Mancuso P, Gobbi A, Pruneri G. The thin red line: angiogenesis in normal and malignant hematopoiesis. Exp Hematol, 28: 993-1000, 2000.
4. de Bont ES, Guikema JE, Scherpen F, Meeuwsen T, Kamps WA, Vellenga E, Bos NA. Mobilized human CD34+ hematopoietic stem cells enhance tumor growth in a nonobese diabetic/severe combined immunodeficient mouse model of human non-Hodgkin's lymphoma. Cancer Res, 61: 7654-7659, 2001.

38. Leek RD. The prognostic role of angiogenesis in breast cancer. Anticancer Res, 21: 4325-4331, 2001.
39. MacConmara M, O'Hanlon DM, Kiely MJ, Connolly Y, Jeffers M, Keane FB. An evaluation of the prognostic significance of vascular endothelial growth factor in node positive primary breast carcinoma. Int J Oncol, 20: 717-721, 2002.
40. Gunel N, Akcali Z, Coskun U, Akyol G, Yamac D, Yenidunya S. Prognostic importance of tumor angiogenesis in breast carcinoma with adjuvant chemotherapy. Pathol Res Pract, 198: 7-12, 2002.
41. van 't Veer LJ, Dai H, van de Vijver MJ, He YD, Hart AA, Mao M, Peterse HL, van der Kooy K, Marton MJ, Witteveen AT, Schreiber GJ, Kerkhoven RM, Roberts C, Linsley PS, Bernards R, Friend SH. Gene expression profiling predicts clinical outcome of breast cancer. Nature, 415: 530-536, 2002
42. Guidi AJ, Berry DA, Broadwater G, Helmchen B, Bleiweiss IJ, Budman DR, Henderson IC, Norton L, Hayes DF. Association of angiogenesis and disease outcome in node-positive breast cancer patients treated with adjuvant cyclophosphamide, doxorubicin, and fluorouracil: a Cancer and Leukemia Group B correlative science study from protocols 8541/8869. J Clin Oncol, 20: 732-742, 2002.
43. Mehta R, Kyshtoobayeva A, Kurosaki T, Small EJ, Kim H, Stroup R, McLaren CE, Li KT, Fruehauf JP. Independent association of angiogenesis index with outcome in prostate cancer. Clin Cancer Res, 7: 81-88, 2001.
44. Tas F, Yavuz E, Aydiner A, Saip P, Disci R, Iplikci A, Topuz E. Angiogenesis and p53 protein expression in breast cancer: prognostic roles and interrelationships. Am J Clin Oncol, 23: 546-553, 2000.
45. Adams J, Carder PJ, Downey S, Forbes MA, MacLennan K, Allgar V, Kaufman S, Hallam S, Bicknell R, Walker JJ, Cairnduff F, Selby PJ, Perren TJ, Lansdown M, Banks RE. Vascular endothelial growth factor (VEGF) in breast cancer: comparison of plasma, serum, and tissue VEGF and microvessel density and effects of tamoxifen. Cancer Res, 60: 2898-2905, 2002.
46. Magennis DP. Angiogenesis: a new prognostic marker for breast cancer. Br J Biomed Sci, 55: 214-220, 1998.
47. Gasparini G, Toi M, Verderio P, Ranieri G, Dante S, Bonoldi E, Boracchi P, Fanelli M, Tominaga T. Prognostic significance of p53, angiogenesis, and other conventional features in operable breast cancer: subanalysis in node-positive and node-negative patients. Int J Oncol, 12: 1117-1125, 1998.
48. Weidner N. Tumoral vascularity as a prognostic factor in cancer patients: the evidence continues to grow. J Pathol, 184: 119-122, 1998.
49. Obermair A, Kucera E, Mayerhofer K, Speiser P, Seifert M, Czerwenka K, Kaider A, Leodolter S, Kainz C, Zeillinger R. Vascular endothelial growth factor (VEGF) in human breast cancer: correlation with disease-free survival. Int J Cancer, 74: 455-458, 1997.
50. Semenza GL. Angiogenesis in ischemic and neoplastic disorders. Annu Rev Med, 54: 17-28, 2003.
51. Liu W, Ahmad SA, Reinmuth N, Shaheen RM, Jung YD, Fan F, Ellis LM. Endothelial cell survival and apoptosis in the tumor vasculature. Apoptosis, 5: 323-328, 2000.
52. Gunsilius E. Evidence from a leukemia model for maintenance of vascular endothelium by bone-marrow-derived endothelial cells. Adv Exp Med Biol, 522: 17-24, 2003.

53. Tsai PW, Shiah SG, Lin MT, Wu CW, Kuo ML. Up-regulation of vascular endothelial growth factor C in breast cancer cells by heregulin-beta 1. A critical role of p38/nuclear factor-kappa B signaling pathway. J Biol Chem, 278: 5750-5759, 2003.
54. Mattila MM, Ruohola JK, Karpanen T, Jackson DG, Alitalo K, Harkonen PL. VEGF-C induced lymphangiogenesis is associated with lymph node metastasis in orthotopic MCF-7 tumors. Int J Cancer, 98: 946-951, 2002.
55. Kinoshita J, Kitamura K, Kabashima A, Saeki H, Tanaka S, Sugimachi K. Clinical significance of vascular endothelial growth factor-C (VEGF-C) in breast cancer. Breast Cancer Res Treat, 66: 159-164, 2001.
56. Skobe M, Hawighorst T, Jackson DG, Prevo R, Janes L, Velasco P, Riccardi L, Alitalo K, Claffey K, Detmar M. Induction of tumor lymphangiogenesis by VEGF-C promotes breast cancer metastasis. Nat Med, 7: 192-198, 2001
57. Gunningham SP, Currie MJ, Han C, Robinson BA, Scott PA, Harris AL, Fox SB. The short form of the alternatively spliced flt-4 but not its ligand vascular endothelial growth factor C is related to lymph node metastasis in human breast cancers. Clin Cancer Res, 6: 4278-4286, 2000.
58. Ruohola JK, Valve EM, Karkkainen MJ, Joukov V, Alitalo K, Harkonen PL. Vascular endothelial growth factors are differentially regulated by steroid hormones and antiestrogens in breast cancer cells. Mol Cell Endocrinol, 149: 29-40, 1999.
59. Joukov V, Sorsa T, Kumar V, Jeltsch M, Claesson-Welsh L, Cao Y, Saksela O, Kalkkinen N, Alitalo K. Proteolytic processing regulates receptor specificity and activity of VEGF-C. EMBO J, 16: 3898-3911, 1997.
60. Kaipainen A, Korhonen J, Mustonen T, van Hinsbergh VWM, Fang GH, Dumont D, Breitman M, Alitalo K. Expression of the fms-like tyrosine kinase FLT4 gene becomes restricted to lymphatic endothelium during development. Proc Natl Acad Sci USA, 92: 3566-3570, 1995.
61. Enholm B, Paavonen K, Ristimaki A, Kumar V, Gunji Y, Klefstrom J, Kivinen L, Laiho M, Olofsson B, Joukov V, Eriksson U, Alitalo K. Comparison of VEGF, VEGF-B, VEGF-C and Ang-1 mRNA regulation by serum, growth factors, oncoproteins and hypoxia. Oncogene, 14: 2475-2483, 1997.
62. Achen M, Jeltsch M, Kukk E, Makinen T, Vitali A, Wilks A, Alitalo K, Stacker SA. Vascular endothelial growth factor D (VEGF-D) is a ligand for the tyrosine kinases VEGF receptor 2 (Flk1) and VEGF receptor 3 (Flt4). Proc Natl Acad Sci USA, 95: 548-553, 1998.
63. Achen MG, Williams RA, Baldwin ME, Lai P, Roufail S, Alitalo K, Stacker SA. The angiogenic and lymphangiogenic factor vascular endothelial growth factor-D exhibits a paracrine mode of action in cancer. Growth Factors, 20: 99-107, 2002.
64. Kurebayashi J, Otsuki T, Kunisue H, Mikami Y, Tanaka K, Yamamoto S, Sonoo H. Expression of vascular endothelial growth factor (VEGF) family members in breast cancer. Jpn J Cancer Res, 90: 977-981, 1999.
65. van der Pluijm G, Lowik C, Papapoulos S. Tumor progression and angiogenesis in bone metastasis from breast cancer: new approaches to an old problem. Cancer Treat Rev, 26: 11-27, 2000.
66. van der Pluijm G, Sijmons B, Vloedgraven H, Deckers M, Papapoulos S, Lowik C. Monitoring metastatic behavior of human tumor cells in mice with species-specific

disease or treatment of the disease including urinary obstruction, loss of sexual function and psychosocial aspects of the disease in early stage prostate cancer patients' and bone pain, osteoporosis and dementia in advanced prostate cancer patients (16, 17). Thus, prostate cancer remains a serious health problem in most westernized countries and the treatment and earlier detection of prostate cancer continues to remain a challenge. The development of novel diagnostic and interventional approaches requires extensive pre-clinical evaluation in models of prostate cancer before moving into clinical evaluation. This review summarizes recent progress in establishing models of prostate cancer and their utility as tools for the evaluation of various interventional strategies for the treatment and diagnosis of prostate cancer.

2. BIOLOGICAL PROGRESSION OF PROSTATE CANCER

As with other hormone dependent malignancies like breast, prostate and ovarian cancer, the biological progression of prostate cancer is the result of many events that ultimately lead to the development of highly invasive, hormone refractory metastatic prostate cancer. These include genetic mutations causing the inactivation or silencing of tumor suppressive genes (2, 18). Some of the additional factors which facilitate tumor progression include sex steroids (androgens), growth factors, angiogenic factors, proteases and cytokines (1, 19-22).

Encapsulated primary prostate tumors are rarely associated with mortality. Rather, it is the development of tumor metastases that ultimately results in death. In patients with prostate cancer, metastasis to the bone is frequently observed in advanced disease (23, 24). While skeletal metastases can be of the osteolytic or osteoblastic variety, those observed in patients with prostate cancer are usually of the osteoblastic phenotype (25-28). It is believed that these osteoblastic metastases are the result of cancer cells producing factors that stimulate osteoblast proliferation, differentiation and eventually bone formation (25). The process of metastasis in prostate cancer is similar to other cancer types. Aggressive forms of prostate growing in the site of origin can invade their surrounding tissue by producing proteolytic enzymes, such as urokinase plasminogen activator (uPA) and matrix metalloproteinases (MMPs), which help breakdown the extracellular matrix surrounding the tumor and the basement membrane surrounding tumor-associated blood vessels (ECM) (25,29). Breakdown of the ECM and the basement membrane allows tumor cells to intravasate into the circulation and to disseminate systemically. Cells that reach organs or bone distal to the prostate can then extravasate from the blood vessels into the stroma of the organ. There they begin growing again with the whole process reinitiated, resulting in the development of tumor metastases at multiple sites.

In addition to proteases, there is increasing evidence to indicate that certain growth factors are involved in the stimulation of bone formation that is associated with metastatic prostate tumors. Patients with prostate cancer have increased levels of endothelin-1 (ET-1), which is known to stimulate bone formation and osteoblast proliferation (26, 27). The TGF-ß superfamily as well as the bone morphogenetic proteins (BMPs), namely BMP-2, BM-3, BMP-4 and BMP-6, have also been shown to be stimulators of bone formation (30). Other growth factors that have been shown to be increased in patients with prostate cancer include parathyroid hormone related peptide (PTHrP), fibroblast growth factor (FGF) and platelet derived growth factors (PDGFs) (31-33). Finally, the amino terminal fragment of uPA has also been shown to exhibit mitogenic activity for osteoblasts, whereas the carboxy terminal proteolytic domain of uPA mediates tumor invasiveness and growth factor activation (34-36). Both of these processes may contribute to the pathogenesis of bone metastasis.

3. ROLE OF GROWTH FACTORS IN PROSTATE CANCER

At least 15-20% of patients with malignancy exhibit hypercalcemia which has now been attributed to the production of parathyroid hormone related peptide (PTHrP) by tumor cells (37, 38). While increased PTHrP production is more commonly observed in patients with breast cancer and multiple myeloma, subsets of prostate cancer patients exhibiting hypercalcemia also show high circulating levels of PTHrP (39). An *in vivo* model of prostate cancer over-expressing PTHrP, where it can act as an autocrine growth factor for tumor cells, was developed to demonstrate the role of PTHrP in promoting prostate tumor growth and to evaluate its ability to promote bone resorbing effects in a malignancy which is more commonly associated with an osteoblastic response (40).

The full-length cDNA encoding rat PTHrP was subcloned into a mammalian expression vector. Dunning R3227 Mat Ly Lu cells were stably transfected with vector alone (CTL) or experimental plasmid (PTHrP) to establish Mat Ly Lu-CTL and MatLyLu-PTHrP cells (40,41). Both control and experimental cells were inoculated s.c. into the right flank of Copenhagen rats and tumor volume was measured at timed intervals. Experimental animals receiving MatLyLu-PTHrP cells were found to have significantly larger tumors when compared to control group of animals injected with MatLyLu-CTL cells. When these control and experimental cells were injected into the left ventricle of Copenhagen rats, no difference was observed in the time to development of hind limb paralysis. However, analysis of plasma from these animals showed increased levels of calcium and PTHrP in animals injected with cells over-expressing PTHrP. This hypercalcemic response was found to be more pronounced following intracardiac injection as compared to s.c. inoculation of cells, which may be attributed to the established bone resorbing effects of PTHrP when expressed at the site of experimental skeletal metastases (vertebral column). Histological characterization of lumbar vertebrae from control animals showed mixed osteoblastic and osteolytic lesions. However, vertebrae of animals inoculated with cells over-expressing PTHrP exhibited increased osteolytic activity which is attributed to the bone resorbing effects of PTHrP (Figure 1). Despite the lack of effect of PTHrP on bone metastasis progression, the use of the MatLyLu *in vivo* model has allowed the investigation of the growth factor-like effects of PTHrP on tumor growth and has also provided a model that allows the monitoring of biochemical surrogates (e.g., plasma PTHrP and calcium) to establish efficacy when evaluating experimental therapeutics targeting prostate cancer growth (40, 42).

The role of other growth factors and cytokines in the progression of prostate cancer metastasis to bone is also unclear. Lee et al. tested a panel of bone-associated growth factors and cytokines for their ability to stimulate the proliferation of prostate cancer cell lines isolated from both soft tissue as well as osseous metastases (43). Variable effects were observed with no clear differentiation in response between the tumor lines isolated from soft tissue compared to those isolated from bone metastases. The role of angiogenesis in promoting the metastastic potential of prostate cancer cells has been well elucidated in other cancer types and may be involved in prostate cancer metastasis as well. The onset of angiogenesis is the result of a change in the equilibrium between pro-angiogenic and anti-angiogenic molecules (44). Several pro-angiogenic molecules include VEGF, FGF and PDGF have been implicated in prostate cancer progression (45, 46). PDGF may play an especially important role in the progression of prostate cancer metastasis as demonstrated in a recent study by Uehara et al. (47).

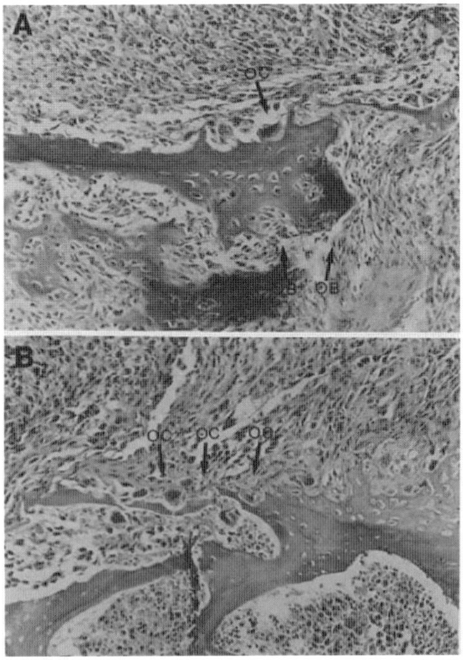

Figure 1. Effect of PTHrP over-expression on skeletal metastases. Male Copenhagen rats were inoculated with MatLyLu (panel A) and MatLyLu-PTHrP cells via intracardiac route of inoculation. At the time of development of hind limb paralysis, animals were sacrificed and histological analysis of lumbar vertebrae from control and experimental animals was carried out. Arrows indicate old bone (OB) and clusters of multinucleated osteoclasts (OC) in areas of bone resorption of experimental animals.

In this study, male athymic mice were injected intra-tibially with a PC-3 cell sub-line (PC-3MM2). Starting at day 3 post tumor cell inoculation, animals were assigned to receive one of four treatment protocols

a) daily dose of vehicle alone;
b) weekly dose of paclitaxel;
c) a daily dose of a known inhibitor of the PDGF receptor, STI 571 (Gleevec) and;
d) a combination of both a weekly dose of paclitaxel and a daily dose of ST1571.

Tumor size and osteolysis of the injected bone were evaluated by digital radiology at the end of the study (47). All of the control animals inoculated with the PC-3MM2 cells and receiving vehicle alone developed osteolytic lesions. While administration of paclitaxel alone had no significant effect on bone lesions, administration of ST1571 alone resulted in a 50% reduction in the number of animals developing osteolytic lesions. Furthermore, the average tumor weight of the lesions in animals receiving either paclitaxel or ST1571 was substantially lower than in control animals receiving vehicle alone (47). The combination of both paclitaxel and ST1571 was the most efficacious treatment in this study, leading to the largest reduction of osteolytic lesions and the lowest tumor weights of all the treatment groups (47). This study implicates the PDGF pathway in the formation and progression of prostate cancer metastasis to bone and provides a validated target that can be evaluated therapeutically in the clinic. This study also emphasizes the probable need for combination therapy approaches for the successful treatment of bone metastasis in patients.

3.1 Role of Proteases in Prostate Cancer

Urikinase Plasminogen Activator (uPA), a member of the serine protease family, is expressed as an enzymatically inactive single chain pro-enzyme (48). Following its activation to the two-chain, enzymatically active form which occurs through limited proteolysis, uPA can activate plasminogen to plasmin, initiating a cascade of events that leads to the activation of several matrix metalloproteases and the release of latent growth factors sequestered to the ECM. Collectively, this chain of events plays a major role in tumor progression. Additionally, the uPA cascade also leads to the degradation and remodeling of the tumor ECM through its effects on laminin, fibronectin, fibrin and collagen (36, 48). This facilitates the intravasation of tumor cells into blood vessels and metastases to distant organs. Finally, uPA plays a major role in promoting the invasive and metastic behaviour of several malignances by directly promoting cell growth, migration and angiogenesis, inducing signals mediated by its specific cell-surface receptor, uPAR (49).

In order to directly establish the role of uPA in prostate cancer progression and metastasis, a syngeneic model of rat prostate cancer was established. MatLyLu rat prostatic carcinoma cells were transfected using experimental plasmids containing rat uPA in both sense and anti-sense orientations (35). This model was established to overcome the issue of species specificity as human uPA fails to bind effectively to rat uPAR and vice versa. Since uPA and uPAR are expressed not only by tumor cells but also by angiogenic endothelial cells and tumor associated macrophages, only a syngeneic or allogeneic model would allow for the full complement of possible uPA-uPAR interactions within a tumor to occur. Control groups of rats inoculated in the left ventricle with untransfected MatLyLu cells routinely developed hind limb paralysis by day 21 post inoculation (35). In contrast, animals receiving Mat Ly Lu cells transfected with the sense uPA vector (MatLyLu-uPA-S) developed paralysis by day 14 whereas the animals inoculated with the anti-sense uPA MatLyLu cells (MatLyLu-uPA-

AS), which expressed lower levels of uPA than the MatLyLu cells transfected with vector alone (MatLyLu- PYN), did not develop hind limb paralysis until day 27 (Figure 2).

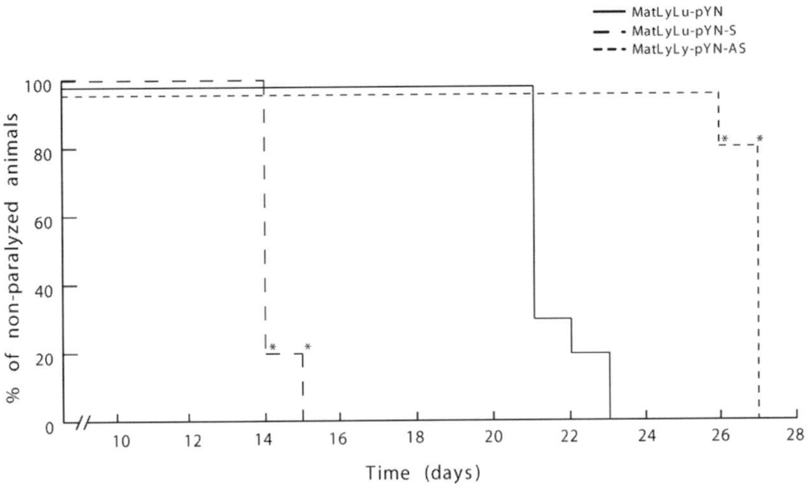

Figure 2. Effect of uPA production on the development of hind limb paralysis. Male Copenhagen rats were inoculated with MatLyLu cells transfected with vector alone (MatLyLu-PYN) or uPA cDNA in anti-sense (MatLyLu-YN-uPA-AS) or sense (MatLyLu-PYN-uPA-S) orientation. The percentage of animals developing hind limb paralysis in each group at various time points was compared. Significant differences from control (MatLyLu-PYN) is shown by asterisks (P<0.05).

Our previous studies had shown that uPA as well as its catalytically inactive amino-terminal fragment were mitogenic for cells of the osteoblastic phenotype *in vitro* and the MatLyLu model allowed us to evaluate the ability of uPA to act as selective mitogen for cells of the osteoblastic phenotype *in vivo* in the context of bone metastasis progression (35). Rats inoculated with parental MatLyLu cells commonly exhibited both osteoblastic and osteolytic lesions. However, animals inoculated with MatLyLu-uPA-S (uPA over-expressing) cells demonstrated a predominantly osteoblastic response in their bone metastases (observed using histological analysis and measurement of serum alkaline phosphatase), effects that were attributed to the mitogenic effects of uPA for cells of the osteoblastic phenotype (Figure 3A). In addition, the serum from control and experimental animals was tested for any change in biochemical parameters associated with increased bone turnover. Experimental animals receiving MatLyLu-uPA-S cells showed increased levels of serum alkaline phosphatase compared to the control group of animals inoculated with MatLyLu-PYN cells (Figure 3B).

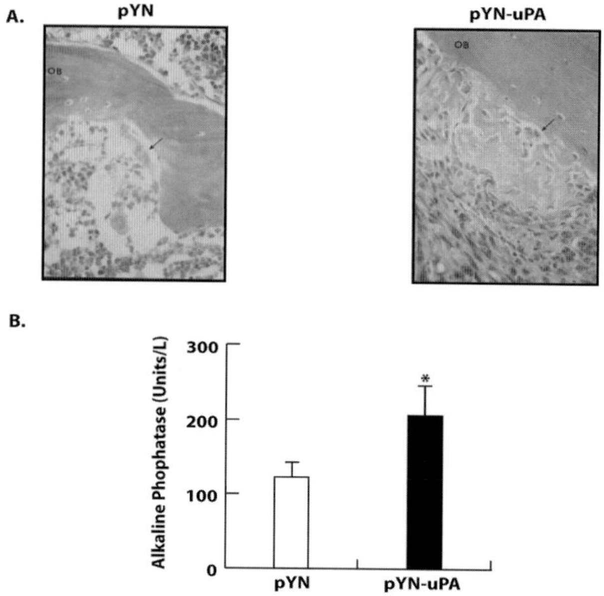

Figure 3. Effect of uPA production on bone turnover. **A**: Light micrograph of lumbar vertebrae of animals inoculated with MatLyLu cells transfected with vector alone (PYN) or cDNA encoding uPA in sense orientation (PYN-uPA). Areas of old bone (OB) and multinucleated osteoclasts in control (PYN) and incrased osteoblastic activity in (PYN-uPA) each group of animals is indicated. **B**: Serum from control (PYN) and experimental (PYN-uPA) animals was analyzed for the level of alkaline phosphatase at the time of developing hind limb paralysis. Significant difference from control is shown by asterisks ($P<0.05$).

Detailed analysis of control and experimental animals also showed that control MatLyLu-PYN animals developed tumor metastases to adrenals, kidney, lungs in addition to skeletal metastases to the lumbar vertebra. Animals receiving MatLyLu-uPA-S routinely developed significantly greater numbers and size of tumor metastases to soft tissues. Additionally these animals not only developed metastases at lumbar vertebrae L1-L2 at a much earlier time period than control animals but also exhibited the presence of skeletal metastases at additional sites (scapula, femur and ribs) (Table 1). Collectively, these studies provide evidence for the role of uPA in tumor cell colonization to skeleton as well as a model for the evaluation of therapeutic strategies targeting the uPA system (35, 36).

Table 1. Assessment of tumor metastases in control and experimental animals. At the time of sacrifice male Copenhagen rats receiving MatLyLu cells transfected with vector alone (MatLyLu-PYN) or uPA (MatLyLu-uPA). Total number of macroscopic metastatic foci at different sites in each group is indicated.

Site of Tumor Metastases	MatLyLu-PYN	MatLyLu-PYN-uPA
Adrenals	2	4
Kidneys	1	3
Lungs	1	2
Vertebral Column	2	4
Scapula	-	2
Ribs	-	2
Femur	-	1

4. MODELS OF PROSTATE CANCER

In order to establish the role of various growth factors and proteases in the multi-step process of prostate cancer progression as well as to evaluate experimental therapeutics, suitable *in vivo* models are needed which best mimic the natural behavior of human prostate cancer. Although this has been a major objective in prostate cancer research for many years and the issue of suitable models has been addressed in various workgroups and publications, the search for suitable models of prostate cancer progression continues (50-52). Human prostate cancer starts as a local non-invasive androgen sensitive disease that may be indolent for some amount of time and may slowly progress into highly invasive, hormone insensitive disease. This progression has been difficult to model in any one single or combination of models. Thus, while several *in vivo* models of prostate cancer are available, continued efforts are needed to develop representative models of human disease. In these models, one would desire reproducibility and progression of disease including invasive behavior and vascular and lymphatic spread to distant organs including bone, where tumor cells can effectively proliferate in the microenvironment of the bone. This is particularly important since tumor or bone derived factors can interact co-operatively in an autocrine or paracrine manner to progressively promote local tumor growth as well as tumor invasion and metastasis to unaffected sites as is often seen in human prostate cancer over time. Prostate cancer can also develop spontaneously in dogs, cats, rats and transgenic mice, which can serve as suitable models for study of this disease. However, these animal models do not develop metastasis and thus, the study of metastasis has been restricted to artificial experimental systems.

4.1 Transgenic Models

While several transplantable models of prostate cancer are commonly used for evaluating experimental therapeutics *in vivo*, autochthonous models have also contributed significantly to our understanding of prostate cancer pathobiology. Use of transgenic and knock out technology in these models has provided a unique opportunity to investigate the significance of a particular gene in the complex process of tumor initiation and progression (53). The transgenic adenocarcinoma of the mouse prostate (TRAMP) has been used effectively to study the role of peptide growth factors in prostate cancer (54, 55). In this well-characterized system, several important features of prostate cancer have been observed including progression from hormone dependence to hormone independence and metastasis to distal organs. This model also allowed investigators to obtain genetic and biochemical information on prostate cancer progression while continuing to maintain an intact immune system. Unfortunately, the TRAMP model is limited due to a lack of representative markers of prostate cancer progression in mice. For example, mice do not express prostate specific antigen (PSA), which makes it difficult to follow disease progression in this host. However, with emerging technologies such as inducible knock-in and knock-out mice, continued progress is being made to develop models that more accurately reproduce human prostate cancer (56, 57). These inducible gene expression systems combined with new state of the art imaging technologies will provide better insight into the development and progression of this disease. Ultimately, newly developed models may become the gold standard for evaluating novel prostate cancer therapeutics but until then, the study of prostate cancer progression and the evaluation of new drugs with the potential for treating prostate cancer will continue to be carried out using existing transplantable prostate cancer models. We will therefore discuss the most commonly used syngeneic and xenograft models of prostate cancer and their utility for studying mechanisms of prostate cancer progression as well as for evaluating novel therapeutic approaches.

4.2 Syngeneic Models of Prostate Cancer

Syngeneic models have several advantages over xenograft models of cancer: there are no species barriers to overcome, since both tumor line and host are derived from the same species; the host is immunocompetent; and tumor take rate and growth are extremely efficient since the tumor line is put back into the same strain of animal from which it was derived, making rejection unlikely. Indeed, numerous tumor lines have been developed from syngeneic systems. For prostate cancer, one of the most frequently used model systems is the Dunning R3227 rat prostate cancer cell line (41). This line was originally identified as a spontaneous adenocarcinoma of the prostate and was found to be slow growing and non-metastatic. However, the isolation of the parental R3227 cell line has led to the establishment of numerous sub-clones with various properties (41). These include the slow-growing, hormone sensitive, androgen receptor positive cell line R3227H and the hormone insensitive, androgen receptor negative, highly invasive R3227AT cell lines. Due to the ability of the R3227AT cells to metastasize to lymph nodes and lungs when implanted into syngeneic hosts (male Copenhagen rats), this line is also referred to as Dunning R3227 – Mat Ly Lu rat prostate cancer cell line (58-61). Since these cell lines represent different stages of prostate cancer progression (from hormone sensitive to hormone insensitive), they have frequently been used to assess the contribution of a gene of interest to the development of prostate cancer as well as for evaluating anti-tumor response to hormonal and bio-therapeutic agents. Apart from the Dunning R3227 parental and sub-cloned cell lines, other less frequently used models of rat prostate cancer including the Lobund-Wistar (L-W) rat and the Wistar-Unilever (WU) rat have been developed (62-65). In the L-W rat model, animals develop spontaneous tumors in the anterior prostate, possibly due to high circulating levels of testosterone. Early stage tumors are hormone dependent for their growth but do become hormone independent as the tumors progress and ~30% of animals will develop metastatic disease (66, 67). This model has been used to test the effect of various interventions on prostate cancer development and has demonstrated the inhibitory effect of diverse approaches such as dietary testosterone ablation, tamoxifen and vitamin D analogues on prostate cancer growth (68, 69). Unfortunately, similar to transgenic models of prostate cancer, the L-W rat is not practical for testing drugs with potential activity against prostate cancer. The spontaneous tumors take a long time to form and it takes ~25 months to develop the most aggressive form of the disease. It would also be difficult to evaluate the effect of a drug on survival in this model since the animals that develop aggressive disease are already very old and will most likely die from something other than cancer before an effect on survival could be observed. The WU model is a hormone dependant prostate cancer model that does not progress to metastatic or hormone insensitive disease and really lends itself to chemoprevention and tumorigenesis studies only. Cell lines developed from L-W rats include PAIII. These cells, when injected close to bone, have been reported to cause a mixed osteoblastic and osteolytic response (70).

MatLyLu cells have been particularly useful for target validation and therapeutic intervention studies (35, 40, 42). Following subcutaneous inoculation of these tumor cells into Copenhagen rats, palpable primary tumors develop by day seven post tumor cell inoculation. These tumors continue to grow in size and lead to tumor metastasis to lungs and lymph nodes which can be readily detected and quantitated by approximately day 18-20, when these animals are sacrificed. Since its development, various Dunning R3227 models of rat prostate cancer have been extensively used for the development and validation of new therapeutic approaches for hormone responsive and hormone refractory prostate cancer. A lytic peptide was tested for its capacity to reduce primary tumor growth and metastases. This peptide was found to be an effective anti-tumor agent in both androgen receptor positive (G) and negative (MatLyLu) Dunning R3227 cells without exhibiting any noticeable side effects on tumor bearing animals (58-60, 71). In another orientation of this model, it is possible to establish experimental metastases to bone by injection of tumor cells into the left ventricle of a rat. These metastases continue to grow in size over the period of 2-3 weeks, eventually causing spinal cord compression and hind limb paralysis (35). The endpoint of this model is easily observed when the animals begin to drag their hind limbs and gives a readout of drug efficacy even before animals are euthanized. Autopsy of these animals also routinely shows distended urinary bladders as well as occasional metastasis to the adrenal glands. Additional details of the experimental metastasis model using Mat Ly Lu cells are discussed in the section titled Role of Proteases in Prostate Cancer.

Production of tumor derived factors at the site of bone metastases has a direct impact on bone turnover. These factors can either act directly or by their ability to activate latent growth factors. These effects are localized within the tumor or bone derived cells where selective receptors for these factors are expressed to direct osteoblastic or ostelytic response. Notable among these are uPA with selective mitogenic effects for osteoblasts, localization of ET-1 due to expression of its receptor on osteoblasts and osteoblast specific transcription factor *Cfba1* which has been implicated in osteoblast differentiation during development and also in bone formation (72, 73).

4.3 Xenograft Models of Prostate Cancer

Although syngeneic animal models provide an excellent opportunity for the evaluation of potential novel therapeutic modalities for prostate cancer, representative models of human origin that mimic the clinical process of the disease are essential to validate these new concepts for potential testing in humans. The introduction of immunodeficient mice such as nude and scid as hosts for xenograft implantation of human prostate cancer opened a new era of cancer research. Unfortunately, the limited availability of experimental model systems has hampered human prostate cancer research for quite a number of years. The lack of representative models was due to the poor growth potential of the implanted human prostate cancer cells/tissues as well as the fact that many of the early prostate cancer cell lines (PC-3, LNCaP, DU145) lacked many of the features of human prostate cancer progression (74). However, in recent years, additional human prostate cancer lines more closely resembling the characteristics found in human prostate cancer have been identified and established. Tumor lines such as CWR22 and CWR22R, LuCaP, RC-9, MDA, VCaP and C4-2 have demonstrated improved tumor takes, spontaneous metastasis and have become increasingly more prominent in the study of prostate cancer progression as well as in the evaluation of novel interventional strategies (75-78). To date, approximately 25 xenograft models of prostate cancer have been established. The available xenograft models represent various stages of the disease ranging from early stage, non-invasive prostate cancer to late stage, highly invasive prostate cancer.

Early stage, well encapsulated prostatic tumors are curable by surgical removal of the tumor mass (79). However the majority of patients diagnosed with prostate cancer have some degree of soft tissue and skeletal metastases which ultimately leads to the high degree of mortality seen among prostate cancer patients (80). Due to the limited therapeutic modalities available to combat this disease at its hormone independent, highly invasive state, sublines of the human prostate cancer PC-3 cells have been used to develop and validate appropriate therapeutic modalities. Several methods of inoculation have been reported and they include s.c., i.c. and orthotopic injections into the long bones or the prostate gland itself. Several human prostate cancer cells lines can also be injected subcutaneously into the right flank of male nude mice which results in the growth of primary tumors that grow and develop systemic metastases to soft tissues such as lungs (81). Although very convenient for the measurement of primary tumors, this model has a major disadvantage of having a high degree of irreproducibility. A more reliable and highly reproducible method involves the orthotopic injection of prostate cancer cells directly into the prostate of mouse (82). This model has been shown to result in rapid local tumor growth with a high rate of soft tissue metastases.

Intracardiac injection of human prostate cancer cells into the left ventricle of nude mice results in bone metastases. This model has many advantages including the testing of Paget's "seed and soil" theory where the cancer cells serve as the "seeds" and the bone microenvironment serves as the "soil" (83, 84). One of the disadvantages of using such a system is the uncertainty in the pathogenesis of the resulting bone metastases after the cells have been injected into the left ventricle. The metastases occur at sites of active bone remodeling, in young mice, with the majority of metastases occurring at the metaphysis of the long bones due to the high number of blood vessels at these sites. The unique anatomical arrangement of the blood vessels in this region provides for common embolism sites (e.g., sites where the injected tumor cells will aggregate) leading to the development of bone metastases in growing rodents.

Human prostate cancer cells can also be injected into the tibia of nude mice. Although more recently developed and established, the many advantages that this mode of tumor cell inoculation possesses has established this mode of transplantation as the preferred method for many bone metastases studies. Other than the relative ease of inoculation compared to i.c. injection, several investigators have reported high success rates when injecting PC-3 cells into the tibia of nude mice. Furthermore, the tumors that develop within the tibia are radiologically and histologically similar to those encountered clinically. Unfortunately, due to the experimentally induced nature of the bone metastases, this method cannot be used to study the early metastatic events such as migration, intravasation and extravasation.

During the complex multistep process of tumor progression, prostate cancer is initiated as an androgen-sensitive cancer followed by gradual transition into a highly metastatic and androgen-independent disease that lacks the expression of functional androgen receptors (AR) (85). Studies were carried out evaluating the effect of re-establishing the androgen sensitivity of late stage prostate cancer. Full length cDNA encoding human AR was subcloned into a mammalian expression vector and transfected into human prostate cancer PC-3 cells (PC-3T). Both control PC-3 cells and experimental PC-3T cells were injected subcutaneously into the right flank of male Balb/c (*nu/nu*) mice and animals were monitored for the development of tumors. Control PC-3 animals developed palpable tumors by week 6 post tumor cell inoculation. In contrast to this, there was a significant delay in tumor growth in animals inoculated with androgen sensitive PC-3T cells and palpable tumors were not observed until week 12 post tumor cell inoculation (86). Furthermore, when PC-3T cells were injected into castrated male Balb/c (*nu/nu*) mice, palpable tumors were observed at a much earlier time compared to the non-castrated animals receiving PC-3T cells. In addition, experimental animals inoculated with PC-3T cells exhibited minimal tumor metastases to the lungs as compared to control animals inoculated with parental PC-3 cells (Figure 4). Analysis of tumoral RNA from control and experimental animals showed decreased levels of PTHrP mRNA in PC-3T tumors due to androgen mediated downregulate of PTHrP expression (86). Collectively, these studies demonstrated the ability of sex steroids to regulate the production of growth factors like PTHrP and confirm the role of androgens in prostate cancer progression *in vivo*.

As mentioned previously, the major cause of mortality from prostate cancer is the metastasis of hormone-refractory cells, especially to bone. Several therapeutic modalities targeting bone metastasis have failed to demonstrate regression in the clinical setting (although a decrease in skeletal-related events and palliation of bone pain was observed in a recently published randomized study of Zoledronate (87). Thus, the identification of effective treatments targeting prostate cancer bone metastasis remains a major unmet clinical need.

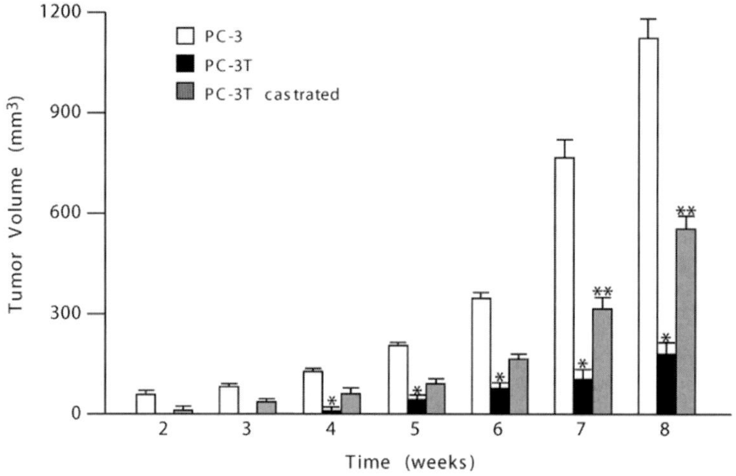

Figure 4. Effect of androgen on prostate tumor cell growth *in vivo*. Human prostate cancer cells PC-3 and cells transfected with androgen receptor (PC-3T) were inoculated into the right flank of normal or castrated male Balb/c mice. Tumor volume was measured at regular intervals. Significant differences in tumor volume from control PC-3 tumor bearing animals is shown by asterisks ($P<0.05$).

4.4 Spontaneous Models of Prostate Cancer in Dogs

Spontaneous prostate cancer in dogs represents a model system that very closely approximates the progression of prostate cancer in man. Prostate cancer occurs most often in elderly, sexually intact dogs or dogs that underwent castration after sexual maturity (88). Most dogs develop adenocarcinoma although the primary tumors tend to appear histologically heterogeneous (89). In a retrospective study of 76 randomly selected dogs with prostate cancer, 80% had metastasis and 22% had metastasis to the bone (88). Those dogs that had bone metastasis demonstrated a predominantly axial skeletal distribution of lesions which is very similar to the distribution of metastases in men with prostate cancer. Therefore, dogs with prostate cancer may offer insight into the progression of prostate cancer in man as well as a system where promising novel therapeutics could be evaluated.

5. EFFICACY OF PROTEASE INHIBITORS IN *IN VIVO* MODELS

Among the various proteases, MMPs are known to play a significant role in the progression of several malignancies including prostate cancer. Thus, the MMP inhibitor A-177430 was evaluated in the MatLyLu model of rat prostate cancer. This new class of MMP inhibitors showed high activity against several key members of MMP family including MMP2 and 9 (90). In Matrigel invasion assays, A-177430 inhibited the invasion of MatLyLu cells through Matrigel in a dose-dependent manner. *In vivo,* A-177430 was infused twice daily at different doses (10 -100 mg/kg) for 15 days following s.c. inoculation of 1 X 10^6 MatLyLu cells. Primary tumor volumes were obtained at timed intervals and animals were sacrificed and evaluated for the presence of macroscopic tumor metastases at day 16 post tumor cell inoculation. These studies demonstrated a dose-dependent effect of A-177430 on reducing primary tumor growth (Figure 5). In addition, while control groups of animals routinely showed large numbers of metastatic tumor foci at lungs, lymph nodes and kidneys, administration of the highest dose of A-177430 (100 mg/kg/day) showed a marked reduction and in some cases, a complete absence of tumor metastases especially in the lungs of experimental animals. The anti-tumor effects of A-177430 were attributed at least partially to the ability of this agent to promote tumor cell apoptosis (Figure 6).

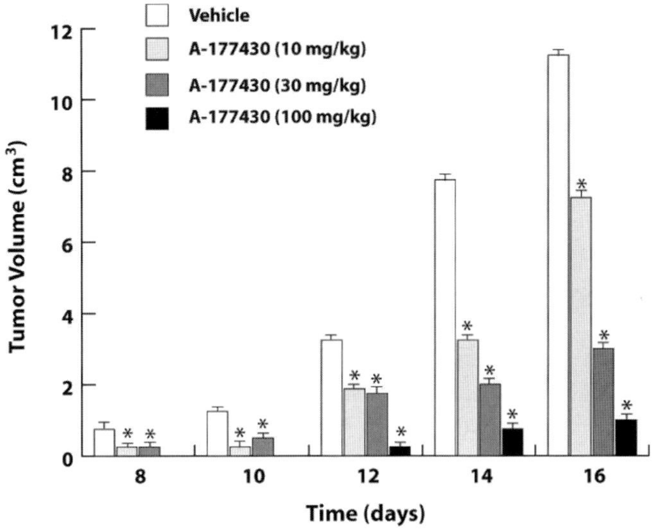

Figure 5. Effect of MMP inhibitor (A-177430) on MatLyLu tumor volume. Male Copenhagen rats inoculated MatLyLu cells (1 X 10^6) into the right flank were treated with vehicle alone or different doses of A-177430. Tumor volume was measured at timed intervals. Significant difference from control is shown by asterisks ($P<0.05$).

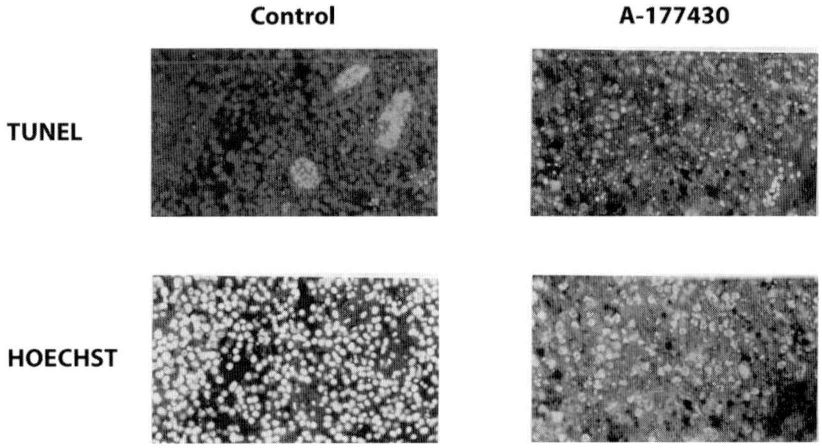

Figure 6. Effect of A-177430 on MatLyLu tumor cell apoptosis *in vivo*. Primary tumors from animals inoculated with MatLyLu cells receiving vehicle alone or A-177430 (100 mg/kg/day) were removed. Following paraffin embedding, sections were processed by TUNEL assay or after TUNEL assay counterstained with Hoechst solution.

The efficacy of a selective inhibitor of uPA (B-428) has also been evaluated in this model. The syngeneic MatLyLu model has been particularly useful in evaluating inhibitors of the uPA system since rat uPA produced by tumor cells was able to fully interact with uPAR expressed by tumor cells and tumor surrounding stromal cells (in contrast to xenograft models, where a species barrier exists to the binding of human uPA to mouse uPAR and vice versa) (91). In addition, the availability of uPA overexpressing tumor cells (MatLyLu-uPA-S) has been useful in establishing highly aggressive models of metastasis. S.c. inoculation of MatLyLu-PYN and MatLyLu-uPA-S cells into Copenhagen rats showed increased tumor growth and metastases in animals receiving MatLyLu-uPA-S. Following s.c. inoculation of these tumor cells, animals were infused with vehicle alone or B-428 (0.24-2.40 mg/kg/day) by implantation of osmotic mini-pumps and tumor volumes were measured at timed intervals. Animals treated with B-428 showed a dose dependent decrease in tumor volume than control group of animals receiving vehicle alone (Figure 7). Finally, a recent study demonstrated that the uPA inhibitor, maspin, could suppress tumor growth, osteolysis and angiogenesis when maspin-overexpressing DU145 cells were injected into human fetal bone fragments implanted in immunodeficient mice (92). Collectively, these results illustrate the central role of the uPA system in prostate cancer progression and validate this system as a therapeutic target for the treatment of prostate cancer.

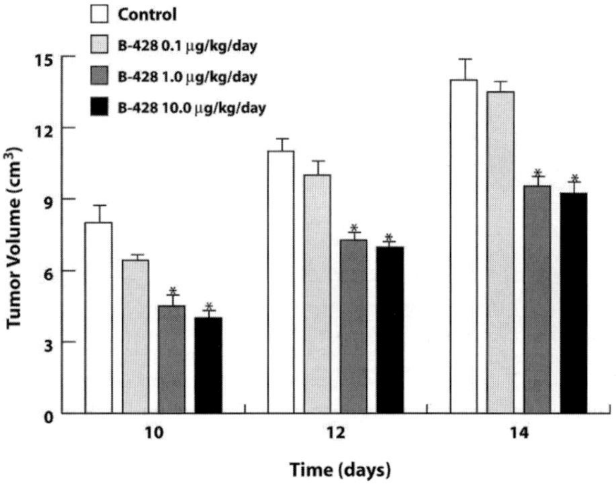

Figure 7. Effect of B-428 on tumor volume. Male Copenhagen rats were inoculated with MatLyLu cells into their right flank. Animals were treated with vehicle alone or B-428 and tumor volume measured at timed intervals. Significant differences from control are shown by asterisks ($P<0.05$).

6. SUMMARY AND CONCLUSIONS

In the past decade, significant improvements and advances have been made in the way prostate cancer is studied in model systems. The advent of novel transgenic and spontaneous models, as well as the establishment of novel cell lines from both spontaneous models and from men with prostate cancer have improved our understanding of the mechanisms responsible for prostate cancer progression. These same models have been used to identify and evaluate novel therapeutic and diagnostic approaches and many of these have been translated into clinical testing. Although many challenges remain, novel high throughput technologies utilizing genomic and proteomic approaches are rapidly changing the way the medical community diagnoses and treats prostate cancer and many of these discoveries are being implemented to more accurately model prostate cancer progression in animals. These improvements will increase our ability to understand prostate cancer progression and ultimately will lead to the development of improved therapeutics for use in this patient population.

REFERENCES

1. Feldman BJ, Feldman D. The development of androgen-independent prostate cancer. Nature Rev Cancer, 1: 34-45, 2001.
2. Kirby RS, Christmas TJ, Brawer MK. *Prostate cancer, second edition,* 2001.
3. Greenlee RT, Hill-Harmon MB, Murray T, Thun M. Cancer statistics. CA Cancer J Clin, 51: 15-36, 2001.
4. Moyad MA. Dietary fat reduction to reduce prostate cancer risk: controlled enthusiasm, learning a lesson from breast or other cancers, and the big picture. Urology, 59: 51-62, 2002.
5. Pollard M, Wolter W, Sun L. Diet and the duration of testosterone-dependent prostate cancer in Lobund-Wistar rats. Cancer Lett, 173: 127-131, 2001.
6. Shi R, Berkel HJ, Yu H. Insulin-like growth factor-1 and prostate cancer: a meta-analysis. Br J Cancer, 85: 991-996, 2001.
7. Chan JM, Giovannucci EL. Diary products, calcium, and vitamin D and risk of prostate cancer. Epidemiol Rev, 23: 87-92, 2001.
8. Pollak M. Insulin-like growth factors and prostate cancer. Epidemiol Rev, 23: 59-66, 2001.
9. Zhang Y, Ni J, Messing EM, Chang E, Yang CR, Yeh S. Vitamin E succinate inhibits the function of androgen receptor and the expression of prostate-specific antigen in prostate cancer cells. Proc Natl Acad Sci USA, 99: 7408-7413, 2002.
10. Yang ES, Maiorino CA, Roos BA, Knight SR, Burnstein KL. Vitamin D-mediated growth inhibition of an androgen-ablated LNCaP cell line model of human prostate cancer. Mol Cell Endocrinol, 186: 69-79, 2002.
11. Fleshner NE. Vitamin E and prostate cancer. Urol. Clin. North Am, 29: 107-113, 2002.

82. Lee C, Shevrin DH, Kozlowski JM. In vivo and in vitro approaches to study metastasis in human prostatic cancer. Cancer Metastasis Rev, 12: 21-28, 1993.
83. Paget S. The distribution of secondary growths in cancer of the breast. Cancer Metastasis Rev, 8: 98-101, 1989.
84. Pettaway CA, Pathak S, Greene G, Ramirez E, Wilson MR, Killion JJ, Fidler IJ. Selection of highly metastatic variants of different human prostatic carcinomas using orthotopic implantation in nude mice. Clin Cancer Res, 2: 1627-1636, 1996.
85. Tilley WD, Wilson CM, Marcelli M, McPhaul MJ. Androgen receptor gene expression in human prostate carcinoma cell lines. Cancer Res, 50: 5382-5386, 1990.
86. Pizzi H, Gladu J, Carpio L, Miao D, Goltzman D, Rabbani SA. Androgen regulation of parathyroid hormone-related peptide production in human prostate cancer cells. Endocrinology, 144: 858-867, 2003.
87. Saad F, Gleason DM, Murray R, Tchekmedyian S, Venner P, Lacombe L, Chin JL, Vinholes JJ, Goas JA, Chen B. A randomized, placebo-controlled trial of zoledronic acid in patients with hormone-refractory metastatic prostate carcinoma. J Natl Cancer Inst, 94:1458-68, 2002.
88. Cornell KK, Bostwick DG, Cooley DM, Hall G, Harvey HJ, Hendrick MJ, Pauli BU, Render JA, Stoica G, Sweet DC, Waters DJ. Clinical and pathologic aspects of spontaneous canine prostate carcinoma: a retrospective analysis of 76 cases. Prostate, 45: 173-183, 2000.
89. Rosol TJ, Tannehill-Gregg SH, LeRoy BE, Mandl S, Contag CH. Animal models of bone metastasis. Cancer, 97(Suppl 3): 748-757, 2003.
90. Rabbani SA, Harakidas P, Guo Y, Steinman D, Davidsen SK, Morgan DW. Synthetic inhibitor of matrix metalloproteases decreases tumor growth and metastases in a syngeneic model of rat prostate cancer in vivo. Int J Cancer, 87: 276-282, 2000.
91. Rabbani SA, Harakidas P, Davidson DJ, Henkin J, Mazar AP. Prevention of prostate-cancer metastasis in vivo by a novel synthetic inhibitor of urokinase-type plasminogen activator (uPA). Int J Cancer, 63: 840-845, 1995.
92. Cher ML, Biliran HR Jr, Bhagat S, Meng Y, Che M, Lockett J, Abrams J, Fridman R, Zachareas M, Sheng S. Maspin expression inhibits osteolysis, tumor growth, and angiogenesis in a model of prostate cancer bone metastasis. Proc Natl Acad Sci. USA, June 3rd, 2003, In Press.

Chapter 10

POTENTIAL THERAPEUTIC TARGETS FOR BONE METASTASIS

Sadmeet Singh and Gurmit Singh
Juravinski Cancer Centre and McMaster University Ontario, Hamilton, Ontario, Canada

1. INTRODUTION

The mortality and morbidity caused by cancer is largely a result of distant spread of the disease. Certain malignancies have a particular propensity to spread to bone amongst which are the three most common cancers – lung, breast and prostate. Patients with lung cancer are more likely to succumb quickly to their disease than those with breast or prostate tumors in whom, relatively, bone metastases are more of a problem. Patients with advanced breast and prostate cancers usually develop bone metastases and tend to harbour the bulk of their tumor burden in their bones at the time of death. The concepts and data reviewed in this chapter relate mainly to these malignancies although some are also relevant to bone metastases secondary to multiple myeloma.

The understanding of molecular mechanisms underlying the pathophysiology of bone metastases is advancing rapidly and as a consequence different processes and steps of the metastatic cascade are being revealed as potential targets for therapy. Increasing numbers of targets are also being identified as a result of the powerful genomic and more recently proteomic screening strategies being employed.

Amongst the phenotypic characteristics of tumors that metastasize to bone are the expression of homing receptors, their associated signaling molecules, extracellular matrix-degrading proteases and other factors responsible for destruction of bone. The influence of the bone environment has long been recognized as a crucial facilitator of bone metastasis and again

G. Singh and W. Orr (eds.), Bone Metastasis and Molecular Mechanisms, 187-210.

a murine osteoblast precursor cell ET-1 has been shown to inhibit differentiation, reduce alkaline phosphatase activity and decrease *in vitro* mineralization (77, 78). These contradictory results may reflect differences in cell lines and ET receptor expression.

In vivo data with breast and prostate cancer cell models support the thesis that ET-1 promotes osteoblastic lesions. Investigators have identified a breast cancer cell line, ZR-75-1, that causes osteoblastic lesions in a mouse model of bone metastases. In contrast to MBA-MB-231 cells which cause osteolytic lesions, analysis of conditioned media from ZR-75-1, cells, was found to contain high levels of ET-1 (79). The conditioned media itself induced new bone formation in mouse calvarial organ cultures as did ET-1. Subsequent *in vivo* experiments have shown that ET_A receptor blockade reduced osteoblastic metastases caused by ZR-75-1 cells but the osteolysis caused by MBA-MB-231 cells was not affected (80). The ET_A receptor antagonist atrasentan (ABT-627) is currently being evaluated in a phase II clinical trial of prostate cancer patients with hormone refractory disease. Initial reports show that markers of bone deposition and resorption are stabilised in patients receiving atrasentan compared to placebo and that these findings were supported by those of clinical bone scan studies (81).

4.2 Stromally Derived Chemokines

The precise mechanisms by which some tumor cells preferentially metastasise to bone remain enigmatic. Three theories are commonly proposed to explain this phenomenon (82). One is that tumor cells leave the circulation in an even distribution across all organs but that they proliferate only in the organs which provide them with the appropriate growth factors. Another is that endothelial cells lining the vessels of the target organs express adhesion molecules that effectively trap the tumor cells. The third theory is one of chemoattraction: tumor cells utilise the chemokine pathway in order to home in on a particular organ such as the bone. Chemokines are similar in structure and function to growth factors. They are produced locally in tissues and bind to G-protein coupled receptors on leukocytes whose migration they are largely responsible for controlling (83). Stimulation of these receptors by chemokines induces the upregulation and activation of integrins enabling leukocytes to adhere to the vascular endothelial cells before migrating into tissues. The similarity in the behaviour of metastasising tumor cells led investigators to test the hypothesis that breast cancer cells express receptors that are activated by the same chemokines (84). They found that the chemokine receptors CXCR4 and CCR7 were highly expressed in breast cancer cells, malignant breast tumors and metastases. The chemokine ligands of these receptors, CXCL12/SDF-1 and

CCL21/6Ckine, were found to be preferentially expressed by tissues to which breast cancer commonly metastasizes: lymph nodes, lung, liver and bone marrow. Markedly lower expression was observed in skin, brain, kidney and skeletal muscle. They went on to show that in a mouse model of breast cancer metastasis, treatment with neutralizing antibodies to CXCR4 impaired the development of lung metastases.

This work has been supported by *in vitro* studies showing that prostate cancer cell lines express high levels of CXCR4 and that osteoblastic cell lines express high levels of SDF-1 (85). In order to assess whether chemokine activity might be involved in bone metastasis in prostate cancer, cells were treated with SDF-1 and found to adhere and migrate preferentially towards bone endothelial cells. *In vitro* invasion of prostate cancer cells was stimulated by SDF-1 but inhibited by CXCR4 antibodies. The expression of CXCR4 has also now been verified in clinical samples of prostate cancer by tissue microarray. CXCL12 mRNA was also detected at higher levels in metastatic than normal tissue (86). The involvement of chemokines in tumor biology is a rapidly advancing field of study (87) and the data reviewed here implies that they are critical regulators of metastasis to bone. Small molecule antagonists of chemokine receptors, under development for a variety of applications (88, 89), represent an attractive means of preventing or treating metastatic bone disease.

4.3 Macrophage Inflammatory Protein –1α

Macrophage inflammatory protein-1α (MIP-1α) is a potent stimulator of osteoclast activity and has recently been identified as mediator of osteolysis in myeloma. Recent data from *in vivo* experiments (90) have confirmed *in vitro* findings that MIP-1α stimulates osteoclast differentiation and bone resorption (91, 92). It is expressed in 70% of patient derived myeloma cells and at much higher concentrations in the supernatants of bone marrow from myeloma patients than those with other haematological malignancies or controls (93). Implantation of a myeloma derived cell line, ARH-77, into SCID mice, causes the animals to develop the clinical features of myeloma including osteolytic lesions and bone destruction. ARH-77 cells expressing an antisense construct to MIP-1α resulted in decreased tumor growth within bone marrow (93). In another mouse model of myeloma, utilising 5TGM1 cells, systemic treatment of animals with an antibody to MIP-1α led to decreased disease progression with significant decreases in bone tumor volume (90). The 5TGM1 cells used express the chemokine receptors CCR1 and CCR5, for which MIP-1α is a ligand (94). These and other chemokine receptors seem to be implicated in the migration and homing mechanisms of myeloma cells to bone. This again offers the opportunity of targeting the

40. Gazitt Y. TRAIL is a potent inducer of apoptosis in myeloma cells derived from multiple myeloma patients and is not cytotoxic to hematopoietic stem cells. Leukemia, 13: 1817-1824, 1999.
41. Oyajobi BO, Anderson DM, Traianedes K, Williams PJ, Yoneda T, Mundy GR. Therapeutic efficacy of a soluble receptor activator of nuclear factor kappaB-IgG Fc fusion protein in suppressing bone resorption and hypercalcemia in a model of humoral hypercalcemia of malignancy. Cancer Res, 61: 2572-2578, 2001.
42. Coleman RE. Metastatic bone disease: clinical features, pathophysiology and treatment strategies. Cancer Treat Rev, 27: 165-176, 2001.
43. Neville-Webbe HL, Holen I, Coleman RE. The anti-tumor activity of bisphosphonates. Cancer Treat Rev, 28: 305-319, 2002.
44. Sidenius N, Blasi F. The urokinase plasminogen activator system in cancer: recent advances and implication for prognosis and therapy. Cancer Metastasis Rev, 22: 205-222, 2003.
45. Hart CA, Scott LJ, Bagley S, Bryden AA, Clarke NW, Lang SH. Role of proteolytic enzymes in human prostate bone metastasis formation: in vivo and in vitro studies. Br J Cancer, 86: 1136-1142, 2002.
46. Fisher JL, Field CL, Zhou H, Harris TL, Henderson MA, Choong PF. Urokinase plasminogen activator system gene expression is increased in human breast carcinoma and its bone metastases--a comparison of normal breast tissue, non-invasive and invasive carcinoma and osseous metastases. Breast Cancer Res Treat, 61: 1-12, 2000.
47. Littlewood-Evans AJ, Bilbe G, Bowler WB, Farley D, Wlodarski B, Kokubo T, Inaoka T, Sloane J, Evans DB, Gallagher JA. The osteoclast-associated protease cathepsin K is expressed in human breast carcinoma. Cancer Res, 57: 5386-5390, 1997.
48. Ishikawa T, Kamiyama M, Tani-Ishii N, Suzuki H, Ichikawa Y, Hamaguchi Y, Momiyama N, Shimada H. Inhibition of osteoclast differentiation and bone resorption by cathepsin K antisense oligonucleotides. Mol Carcinog, 32: 84-91, 2001.
49. McCawley LJ, Matrisian LM. Matrix metalloproteinases: they're not just for matrix anymore! Curr Opin Cell Biol, 13: 534-540, 2001.
50. Everts V, Delaisse JM, Korper W, Beertsen W. Cysteine proteinases and matrix metalloproteinases play distinct roles in the subosteoclastic resorption zone. J Bone Min Res, 13: 1420-1430, 1998.
51. Lhotak S, Elavathil LJ, Vukmirovic-Popovic S, Duivenvoorden WC, Tozer RG, Singh G. Immunolocalization of matrix metalloproteinases and their inhibitors in clinical specimens of bone metastasis from breast carcinoma. Clin Exp Metastasis, 18: 463-470, 2000.
52. Coussens LM, Fingleton B, Matrisian LM. Matrix metalloproteinase inhibitors and cancer: trials and tribulations. Science, 295: 2387-2392, 2002.
53. Overall CM, Lopez-Otin C. Strategies for MMP inhibition in cancer: innovations for the post-trial era. Nat Rev Cancer, 2: 657-672, 2002.
54. Cal S, Obaya AJ, Llamazares M, Garabaya C, Quesada V, Lopez-Otin C. Cloning, expression analysis, and structural characterization of seven novel human ADAMTSs, a family of metalloproteinases with disintegrin and thrombospondin-1 domains. Gene, 283: 49-62, 2002.

55. Blobel CP. Functional and biochemical characterization of ADAMs and their predicted role in protein ectodomain shedding. Inflamm Res, 51: 83-84, 2002.
56. Sanchez-Sweatman OH, Orr FW, Singh G. Human metastatic prostate PC3 cell lines degrade bone using matrix metalloproteinases. Invasion Metastasis, 18: 297-305, 1998.
57. Nemeth JA, Yousif R, Herzog M, Che M, Upadhyay J, Shekarriz B, Bhagat S, Mullins C, Fridman R, Cher ML. Matrix metalloproteinase activity, bone matrix turnover, and tumor cell proliferation in prostate cancer bone metastasis. J Natl Cancer Inst, 94: 17-25, 2002.
58. Falardeau P, Champagne P, Poyet P, Hariton C, Dupont E. Neovastat, a naturally occurring multifunctional antiangiogenic drug, in phase III clinical trials. Semin Oncol, 28: 620-625, 2001.
59. Winding B, NicAmhlaoibh R, Misander H, Hoegh-Andersen P, Andersen TL, Holst-Hansen C, Heegaard AM, Foged NT, Brunner N, Delaisse JM. Synthetic matrix metalloproteinase inhibitors inhibit growth of established breast cancer osteolytic lesions and prolong survival in mice. Clin Cancer Res, 8: 1932-1939, 2002.
60. Golub LM, Lee HM, Lehrer G, Nemiroff A, McNamara TF, Kaplan R, Ramamurthy NS. Minocycline reduces gingival collagenolytic activity during diabetes. Preliminary observations and a proposed new mechanism of action. J Periodontal Res, 18: 516-526, 1983.
61. Golub LM, Lee HM, Ryan ME, Giannobile WV, Payne J, Sorsa T. Tetracyclines inhibit connective tissue breakdown by multiple non-antimicrobial mechanisms. Adv Dent Res, 12: 12-26, 1998.
62. Smith GN Jr, Brandt KD, Hasty KA. Activation of recombinant human neutrophil procollagenase in the presence of doxycycline results in fragmentation of the enzyme and loss of enzyme activity. Arthritis Rheum, 39: 235-244, 1996.
63. Golub LM, Ramamurthy NS, Llavaneras A, Ryan ME, Lee HM, Liu Y, Bain S, Sorsa, T. A chemically modified nonantimicrobial tetracycline (CMT-8) inhibits gingival matrix metalloproteinases, periodontal breakdown, and extra- oral bone loss in ovariectomized rats. Ann NY Acad Sci, 878: 290-310, 1999.
64. Bettany JT, Peet NM, Wolowacz RG, Skerry TM, Grabowski PS. Tetracyclines induce apoptosis in osteoclasts. Bone, 27: 75-80, 2000.
65. Duivenvoorden WC, Hirte HW, Singh G. Use of tetracycline as an inhibitor of matrix metalloproteinase activity secreted by human bone-metastasizing cancer cells. Invasion Metastasis, 17: 312-322, 1997.
66. Fife RS, Sledge GW Jr, Roth BJ, Proctor C. Effects of doxycycline on human prostate cancer cells in vitro. Cancer Lett, 127: 37-41, 1998.
67. Fife RS, Sledge GW Jr. Effects of doxycycline on in vitro growth, migration, and gelatinase activity of breast carcinoma cells. J Lab Clin Med, 125: 407-411, 1995.
68. Fife RS, Sledge GW Jr, Sissons S, Zerler B. Effects of tetracyclines on angiogenesis in vitro. Cancer Lett, 153: 75-78, 2000.
69. Duivenvoorden, WC, Popovic SV, Lhotak S, Seidlitz E, Hirte HW, Tozer RG, Singh G. Doxycycline decreases tumor burden in a bone metastasis model of human breast cancer. Cancer Res, 62: 1588-1591, 2002.
70. Nelson J, Bagnato A, Battistini B, Nisen P. The endothelin axis: emerging role in cancer. Nat Rev Cancer, 3: 110-116, 2003.

71. Stern P H, Tatrai A, Semler DE, Lee SK, Lakatos P, Strieleman PJ, Tarjan G, Sanders JL. Endothelin receptors, second messengers, and actions in bone. J Nutr, 125: 2028S-2032S, 1995.
72. Takuwa Y, Masaki T, Yamashita K. The effects of the endothelin family peptides on cultured osteoblastic cells from rat calvariae. Biochem Biophys Res Commun, 170: 998-1005, 1990.
73. Sasaki T, Hong MH. Endothelin-1 localization in bone cells and vascular endothelial cells in rat bone marrow. Anat Rec, 237: 332-337, 1993.
74. Zaidi M, Alam AS, Bax BE, Shankar VS, Bax CM, Gill JS, Pazianas M, Huang CL, Sahinoglu T, Moonga BS, et al. Role of the endothelial cell in osteoclast control: new perspectives. Bone, 14: 97-102, 1993.
75. Tatrai A, Foster S, Lakatos P, Shankar G, Stern PH. Endothelin-1 actions on resorption, collagen and noncollagen protein synthesis, and phosphatidylinositol turnover in bone organ cultures. Endocrinol, 131: 603-607, 1992.
76. Kasperk CH, Borcsok I, Schairer HU, Schneider U, Nawroth PP, Niethard FU, Ziegler R. Endothelin-1 is a potent regulator of human bone cell metabolism in vitro. Calcif Tissue Int, 60: 368-374, 1997.
77. Takuwa Y, Ohue Y, Takuwa N, Yamashita K. Endothelin-1 activates phospholipase C and mobilizes Ca2+ from extra- and intracellular pools in osteoblastic cells. Am J Physiol, 257: E797-E803, 1989.
78. Hiruma Y, Inoue A, Shiohama A, Otsuka E, Hirose S, Yamaguchi A, Hagiwara H. Endothelins inhibit the mineralization of osteoblastic MC3T3-E1 cells through the A-type endothelin receptor. Am J Physiol, 275: R1099-R1105, 1998.
79. Mundy G, Garrett R, Harris S, Chan J, Chen D, Rossini G, Boyce B, Zhao M, Gutierrez G. Stimulation of bone formation in vitro and in rodents by statins. Science, 286: 1946-1949, 1999.
80. Guise TA, Yin JJ, Mohammad KS. Role of endothelin-1 in osteoblastic bone metastases. Cancer, 97: 779-784, 2003.
81. Carducci MA, Padley RJ, Breul J, Vogelzang NJ, Zonnenberg BA, Daliani DD, Schulman CC, Nabulsi AA, Humerickhouse RA, Weinberg MA, Schmitt JL, Nelson JB. Effect of endothelin-A receptor blockade with atrasentan on tumor progression in men with hormone-refractory prostate cancer: a randomized, phase II, placebo-controlled trial. J Clin Oncol, 21: 679-689, 2003.
82. Liotta LA. An attractive force in metastasis. Nature, 410: 24-25, 2001.
83. Baggiolini M. Chemokines and leukocyte traffic. Nature, 392: 565-568, 1998.
84. Muller A, Homey B, Soto H, Ge N, Catron D, Buchanan ME. Involvement of chemokine receptors in breast cancer metastasis. Nature, 410: 50-56, 2001.
85. Taichman RS, Cooper C, Keller ET, Pienta KJ, Taichman NS, McCauley LK. Use of the stromal cell-derived factor-1/CXCR4 pathway in prostate cancer metastasis to bone. Cancer Res, 62: 1832-1837, 2002.
86. Sun YX, Wang J, Shelburne CE, Lopatin DE, Chinnaiyan AM, Rubin MA, Pienta KJ, Taichman RS. Expression of CXCR4 and CXCL12 (SDF-1) in human prostate cancers (PCa) in vivo. J Cell Biochem, 89: 462-473, 2003.
87. Strieter RM. Chemokines: not just leukocyte chemoattractants in the promotion of cancer. Nat Immunol, 2: 285-286, 2001.

88. Proudfoot AE, Power CA, Wells TN. The strategy of blocking the chemokine system to combat disease. Immunol Rev, 177:246-56, 2000.
89. Rajarathnam K. Designing decoys for chemokine-chemokine receptor interaction. Curr Pharm Des, 8: 2159-2169, 2002.
90. Oyajobi BO, Franchin G, Williams PJ, Pulkrabek D, Gupta A, Munoz S, Grubbs B, Zhao M, Chen D, Sherry B, Mundy GR. Dual effects of macrophage inflammatory protein-1{alpha} on osteolysis and tumor burden in the murine 5TGM1 model of myeloma bone disease. Blood, 102:311-319, 2003.
91. Kukita T, Nomiyama H, Ohmoto Y, Kukita A, Shuto T, Hotokebuchi T, Sugioka Y, Miura R, Iijima T. Macrophage inflammatory protein-1 alpha (LD78) expressed in human bone marrow: its role in regulation of hematopoiesis and osteoclast recruitment. Lab Invest, 76: 399-406, 1997.
92. Han JH, Choi SJ, Kurihara N, Koide M, Oba Y, Roodman GD. Macrophage inflammatory protein-1alpha is an osteoclastogenic factor in myeloma that is independent of receptor activator of nuclear factor kappaB ligand. Blood, 97: 3349-3353, 2001.
93. Choi SJ, Cruz JC, Craig F, Chung H, Devlin RD, Roodman GD, Alsina M. Macrophage inflammatory protein 1-alpha is a potential osteoclast stimulatory factor in multiple myeloma. Blood, 96: 671-675, 2000.
94. Menten P, Wuyts A, van Damme J. Macrophage inflammatory protein-1. Cytokine Growth Factor Rev, 13: 455-481, 2002.
95. De Vos J, Couderc G, Tarte K, Jourdan M, Requirand G, Delteil MC, Rossi JF, Mechti N, Klein B. Identifying intercellular signaling genes expressed in malignant plasma cells by using complementary DNA arrays. Blood, 98: 771-780, 2001.
96. Moller C, Stromberg T, Juremalm M, Nilsson K, Nilsson G. Expression and function of chemokine receptors in human multiple myeloma. Leukemia, 17: 203-210, 2003.
97. Broek IV, Asosingh K, Vanderkerken K, Straetmans N, van Camp B, van Riet I. Chemokine receptor CCR2 is expressed by human multiple myeloma cells and mediates migration to bone marrow stromal cell-produced monocyte chemotactic proteins MCP-1, -2 and -3. Br J Cancer, 88: 855-862, 2003.
98. Nakayama T, Hieshima K, Izawa D, Tatsumi Y, Kanamaru A, Yoshie O. Cutting edge: profile of chemokine receptor expression on human plasma cells accounts for their efficient recruitment to target tissues. J Immunol, 170: 1136 1140, 2003.
99. Heldin CH, Westermark B. Mechanism of action and in vivo role of platelet-derived growth factor. Physiol Rev, 79: 1283-1316, 1999.
100. Yi B, Williams PJ, Niewolna M, Wang Y, Yoneda T. Tumor-derived platelet-derived growth factor-BB plays a critical role in osteosclerotic bone metastasis in an animal model of human breast cancer. Cancer Res, 62: 917-923, 2002.
101. Uehara H, Kim SJ, Karashima T, Shepherd DL, Fan D, Tsan R, Killion JJ, Logothetis C, Mathew P, Fidler IJ. Effects of blocking platelet-derived growth factor-receptor signaling in a mouse model of experimental prostate cancer bone metastases. J Natl Cancer Inst, 95: 458-470, 2003.
102. Druker BJ, Talpaz M, Resta DJ, Peng B, Buchdunger E, Ford JM, Lydon NB, Kantarjian H, Capdeville R, Ohno-Jones S, Sawyers CL. Efficacy and safety of a

specific inhibitor of the BCR-ABL tyrosine kinase in chronic myeloid leukemia. N Engl J Med, 344: 1031-1037, 2001.

103. Buchdunger E, Cioffi CL, Law N, Stover D, Ohno-Jones S, Druker BJ, Lydon NB. Abl protein-tyrosine kinase inhibitor STI571 inhibits in vitro signal transduction mediated by c-kit and platelet-derived growth factor receptors. J Pharmacol Exp Ther, 295: 139-145, 2000.
104. Weber GF. The metastasis gene osteopontin: a candidate target for cancer therapy. Biochim Biophys Acta, 1552: 61-85, 2001.
105. Yeatman TJ, Chambers AF. Osteopontin and colon cancer progression. Clin Exp Metastasis, 20: 85-90, 2003.
106. Furger KA, Menon RK, Tuckl AB, Bramwelll VH, Chambers AF. The functional and clinical roles of osteopontin in cancer and metastasis. Curr Mol Med, 1: 621-632, 2001.
107. Hotte SJ, Winquist EW, Stitt L, Wilson SM, Chambers AF. Plasma osteopontin: associations with survival and metastasis to bone in men with hormone-refractory prostate carcinoma. Cancer, 95: 506-512, 2002.
108. Nemoto H, Rittling SR, Yoshitake H, Furuya K, Amagasa T, Tsuji K, Nifuji A, Denhardt DT, Noda M. Osteopontin deficiency reduces experimental tumor cell metastasis to bone and soft tissues. J Bone Min Res, 16: 652-659, 2001.
109. Pecheur I, Peyruchaud O, Serre CM, Guglielmi J, Voland C, Bourre F, Margue C, Cohen-Solal M, Buffet A, Kieffer N, Clezardin P. Integrin alpha(v)beta3 expression confers on tumor cells a greater propensity to metastasize to bone. FASEB J, 16: 1266-1268, 2002.
110. Liapis H, Flath A, Kitazawa S. Integrin alpha V beta 3 expression by bone-residing breast cancer metastases. Diagn Mol Pathol, 5: 127-135, 1996.
111. Ducy P, Karsenty G. The family of bone morphogenetic proteins. Kidney Int, 57: 2207-2214, 2000.
112. Khan SN, Sandhu HS, Lane JM, Cammisa FP Jr, Girardi FP. Bone morphogenetic proteins: relevance in spine surgery. Orthop Clin North Am, 33: 447-463, ix, 2002.
113. Masuda H, Fukabori Y, Nakano K, Takezawa Y, CSuzuki T, Yamanaka H. Increased expression of bone morphogenetic protein-7 in bone metastatic prostate cancer. Prostate, 54: 268-274, 2003.
114. Thomas BG, Hamdy FC. Bone morphogenetic protein-6: potential mediator of osteoblastic metastases in prostate cancer. Prostate Cancer Prostatic Dis, 3: 283-285, 2000.

Chapter 11

OPG, RANK AND RANKL IN BONE METASTASIS AND CANCER-ASSOCIATED OSTEOLYSIS

Paul J. Kostenuik
Research Scientist, Amgen Inc., Thousand Oaks, California, USA

1. INTRODUCTION

A triad of recently discovered proteins has dominant effects on most aspects of physiological and pathological bone resorption. The discovery of these proteins helped to resolve numerous questions regarding the exact molecular mechanisms for bone resorption. These proteins also neatly account for the long-recognized dependence of osteoclasts on the osteoblast/stromal cell population. This pathway was rapidly elucidated after the discovery of osteoprotegerin (OPG), an endogenous protein that negatively controls most aspects of osteoclast formation, activation and survival. The biological counterpart for OPG is RANKL (receptor activator of nuclear factor-κB ligand), a protein that promotes osteoclast formation, activation and survival. RANKL functions by binding to its receptor RANK on the surface of osteoclasts and their precursors. RANKL is the final mediator of osteoclast activation induced by most, if not all, proresorptive cytokines.

In the simplest terms, bone resorption is initiated by RANKL binding to RANK. Bone resorption is arrested when OPG binds and neutralizes RANKL, thereby preventing the latter from binding to RANK (Figure 1). An important take-home message is that bone resorption is governed by the relative abundance of OPG and RANKL (Figure 2). A relative excess of RANKL leads to bone resorption, while a relative excess of OPG arrests

G. Singh and W. Orr (eds.), Bone Metastasis and Molecular Mechanisms, 211-240

bone resorption. A variety of tumor-derived growth factors and cytokines can influence the expression of OPG and RANKL. The ultimate effect of tumor derived factors on bone resorption cannot be accurately predicted without accounting for changes in the relative abundance of both OPG and RANKL. Most if not all forms of pathologic bone resorption rely on the OPG/RANK/RANKL pathway. Conditions that involve accelerated bone resorption, ranging from rheumatoid arthritis to spaceflight, appear to cause bone loss via this axis. Cancer is among the more common conditions that involve pathological bone loss, and cancer cells have evolved several mechanisms to commandeer the OPG/RANK/RANKL pathway to activate osteoclasts. Some tumors appear to produce their own RANKL to directly activate osteoclasts, while others produce factors that induce RANKL expression by other cells such as osteoblasts and stromal cells. Other tumor types, such as multiple myeloma, may sequester OPG and thereby increase the relative abundance of RANKL.

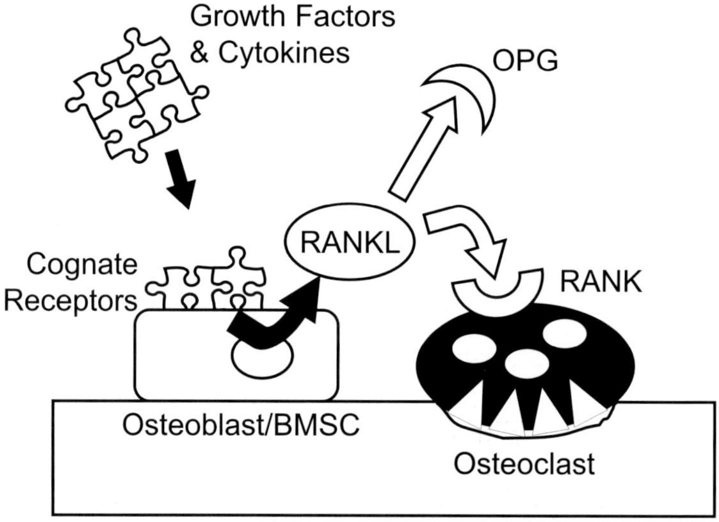

Figure 1. Basic biology of the OPG/RANK/RANKL axis. Various growth factors and cytokines bind to their cognate receptors on osteoblasts or bone marrow stromal cells (BMSCs). Signaling of these receptors may culminate in the production of RANKL. Osteoblasts/BMSCs also produce OPG, a soluble decoy receptor that can bind and neutralize RANKL. If RANKL is not bound by OPG, it is able to bind to RANK on osteoclasts and osteoclast precursors. RANKL binding to RANK causes osteoclast formation, activation and survival, resulting in increased bone resorption.

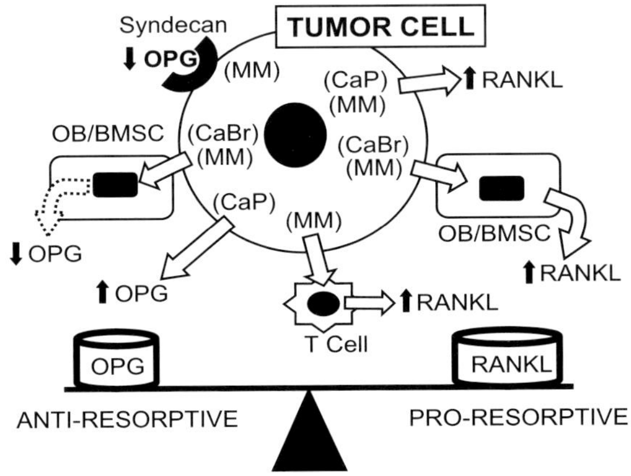

Figure 2. Bone resorption is governed by the relative abundance of OPG (anti-resorptive) and RANKL (pro-resorptive). Tumor cells utilize several mechanisms to upset the balance of OPG and RANKL to favor osteolysis. Clockwise from upper right: Prostate Cancer (CaP) and Multiple Myeloma (MM) cells may produce RANKL directly. Breast Cancer (CaBr) and MM cells may induce RANKL production from osteoblasts and bone marrow stromal cells (BMSC). MM cells may induce T cell production of RANKL. CaP cells can secrete OPG directly, which might serve to inhibit osteolysis. CaBr and MM cells may suppress the production of OPG by osteoblasts and BMSCs. MM cells may bind and degrade OPG via Syndecan-1.

While the OPG/RANK/RANKL axis may neatly account for the mechanisms of osteolysis, the mechanisms responsible for cancer cell osteotropism remain unclear. It was recognized over 100 years ago that breast cancer cells have a special prediliction for bone. Other neoplasms, including multiple myeloma, also have a propensity to spread and grow within the skeleton. The growth of these metastases is usually accompanied by focal osteoclast-mediated osteolysis that can lead to pain, hypercalcemia, immobility and death. The reasons why certain malignancies tend to thrive in bone remain unclear and are likely to be multifactorial. However, a recurring conclusion from animal studies of experimental bone metastasis is that bone resorption often favors skeletal tumor growth. The ability of many bone-metastasizing tumors to increase bone resorption may create a vicious cycle of bone destruction and tumor growth. This chapter will summarize an emerging body of literature that implicates RANKL as a major culprit in this pathological process.

The chapter will first discuss the basic biology of the OPG/RANK/RANKL pathway. Attention will then shift to describing the regulated expression of these proteins in cells and tissues that are associated with bone metastases. Studies that describe the localization and regulation of these proteins have been tremendously informative to our understanding of exacerbate osteolysis, particularly when accompanied by the induction of RANKL. Patients with myeloma had reduced OPG levels in their serum (35, 40) and in bone marrow plasma (41). Myeloma patients with lytic disease also had lower serum OPG levels than those without lytic disease, and lower OPG levels were associated with poorer WHO performance status (42). Serum OPG levels did not however predict treatment response or survival in those patients. Several hypothetical mechanisms have been proposed to explain the decreased OPG levels observed in myeloma patients, and there is little reason to believe that these mechanisms are mutually exclusive. Osteoblasts and stromal cells are major contributors to the OPG pool, and it is possible that myeloma causes reduced OPG production by these cells. In support of this notion, OPG mRNA expression by osteoblasts or stromal cells was suppressed when co-cultured with human myeloma cells (Figure 2) (23, 35). In human bone marrow biopsies, the presence of myeloma was associated with reduced stromal cell and osteoblastic expression of OPG mRNA (23, 35). Serum OPG levels in myeloma patients correlated with a serum marker of bone formation (42), suggesting that a general suppression of osteoblast function in advanced myeloma could lead to reduced OPG production.

Another intriguing hypothesis for reduced OPG levels in myeloma patients is that myeloma cells themselves may bind and sequester OPG (Figure 2). Several myeloma cell lines, as well as primary myeloma cells, have been shown to bind human OPG in tissue culture studies (41, 43). OPG binding to myeloma cell membranes may be mediated by syndecan-1, a transmembrane proteoglycan with heparan sulfate side chains that is expressed on normal and malignant plasma cells (Figure 2) (41). Native OPG has a highly conserved heparin binding domain (7) that is presumably the target for syndecan binding, as OPG binding to syndecan-1 was greatly reduced in the presence of soluble heparin (41). OPG can be rapidly internalized and degraded after binding to cultured myeloma cells, a phenomenon that may contribute to the reduced OPG levels in myeloma patients (41). It remains to be proven whether myeloma cells can directly bind and neutralize OPG in vivo, but it is interesting to note that plasma cells in the bone marrow of myeloma patients stain positive for OPG protein (41). This staining did not appear to result from endogenous OPG production, as myeloma cell lines did not express OPG mRNA or protein (35, 41). It is worth noting that the heparin binding domain of OPG is not necessary for its binding to RANKL (7), and OPG lacking the heparin binding domain did not bind to myeloma cells (43). Therapeutic forms of OPG lack this heparin binding domain, and it is therefore probable that these drugs would avoid the myeloma cell binding and degradation fate while maintaining their antiresorptive potential (44).

3.2 Breast Cancer

Bone metastasis from breast cancer is typically associated with focal osteolysis, and a variety of breast cancer-derived factors have been implicated as osteoclast activating factors (reviewed in 22). Breast cancer cells may be capable of releasing soluble factors that directly activate osteoclasts (45), but it is unlikely that many breast tumors directly produce RANKL. In one study, twelve of twelve primary breast tumors failed to express RANKL mRNA (46), and another study failed to demonstrate RANKL expression by immunohistochemistry (47). Human breast cancer cell lines, including MDA-231, MCF-7 and T47D, fail to express RANKL mRNA (46, 48, 49). The majority of breast cancer-derived factors appear to stimulate osteoclasts indirectly. Before the discovery of OPG/RANKL, it was appreciated that many breast cancer-derived factors act on cells of the osteoblast lineage to induce bone resorption (50). In fact, the presence of osteoblasts or stromal cells is typically required in order for breast cancer cells to induce osteoclastogenesis (46, 51, 52). This requirement may be explained by data from co-culture studies, wherein the presence of breast cancer cells caused osteoblasts or stromal cells to increase their production of RANKL while reducing their production of OPG (Figure 2) (46, 51). This reciprocal control of OPG and RANKL might serve to amplify the pro-resorptive signal by increasing the relative abundance of RANKL. The addition of exogenous OPG to these co-culture systems blocked the ability of breast cancer cells to induce the osteoblast-mediated stimulation of osteoclasts (52).

Breast cancer cells probably secrete a number of pro-resorptive factors that act via osteoblasts and stromal cells, and the best characterized of these factors is PTHrP. PTHrP is frequently produced by human breast cancer cells (53), and tumor-derived PTHrP is a common catalyst for osteolysis and hypercalcemia (54, 55). PTHrP alone is able to mimic many of the activities of breast cancer cells in co-culture models of osteoclastogenesis. For example, PTHrP requires osteoblasts or stromal cells to exert its osteoclastogenic influence (56). The binding of PTHrP to PTH/PTHrP receptors on these cells leads to the stimulation of RANKL (46, 49) and the suppression of OPG (46). PTHrP overexpression by breast cancer cells is sufficient to induce RANKL, suppress OPG, and stimulate osteoclastogenesis in co-cultures that include osteoblasts (46).

Breast cancer-derived PTHrP also appears to use similar mechanisms in vivo to promote osteolysis. In a nude mouse calvarial injection model, the expression of PTHrP by human MCF-7 breast cancer cells was associated with increased RANKL expression by osteoblasts and the induction of bone resorption (49). MCF-7 cells expressing PTHrP were also better able to survive and migrate along the calvarial surface compared to MCF-7 cells that did not produce PTHrP. While PTHrP has a well-defined role in mediating breast cancer-associated osteolysis, the role of PTHrP in promoting bone metastasis and osteotropism is less clear. Elegant studies have supported a causal role for PTHrP in animal models of bone metastasis (57), while data from other studies using similar models have argued against this role (58). Clinical data has suggested that PTHrP production by breast cancer cells is associated with improved survival and reduced bone metastasis (59). While there is a lack of concensus regarding the role for PTHrP in the development of bone metastasis, there is little debate that PTHrP promotes bone resorption through mechanisms that are dependent on OPG/RANK/RANKL (20).

Despite our improved understanding of osteolysis in breast cancer, the mechanisms responsible for breast cancer osteotropism are still poorly understood. Recent observations from RANK knockout mice have provided the basis for a new hypothesis for osteotropism that warrants vigorous testing and challenges. Breast cancer cells frequently express RANK mRNA 46, but the function or consequences of this expression is unknown. Potential clues for RANK function on breast cancer cells are provided by examining the role of RANK in normal mammary epithelial cells, from which most mammary carcinomas arise. The expression of RANK protein is highly restricted (9, 20), so it was somewhat surprising to learn that murine mammary epithelial cells also expressed RANK (60). A functional role for RANK on these cells was strongly supported by observations that mammary gland development during pregnancy was completely arrested in mice lacking RANKL. RANK knockout mice had similar mammary gland defects and were also unable to lactate. Supplementation of RANKL knockout mice with recombinant RANKL rescued the mammary defect, but RANKL supplementation did not rescue the defect in RANK knockout mice. These data indicate that RANK signaling was necessary and sufficient for mammary development during pregnancy (60). RANK was constitutively expressed by mammary epithelial cells, while RANKL was not constitutively expressed but was strongly induced during pregnancy. This induction was associated with alveolar epithelial cell proliferation, avoidance of apoptosis, and ultimately the formation of lobulo-alveolar structures that support lactaction (60). The injection of progesterone, prolactin or PTHrP also induced RANKL expression in mouse mammary tissue, suggesting that these factors may account for the pregnancy-related induction of RANKL.

It is unclear whether the human mammary gland uses similar pathways to regulate lactation during pregnancy. A more provocative question is whether mammary epithelial cells retain functional RANK expression after neoplastic transformation. Early data support this possibility, as RANK mRNA expression was demonstrated in all twelve primary breast cancers analyzed (46). Human breast cancer cell lines also express RANK mRNA (46) (and our unpublished data). The expression of functional RANK protein has been reported in human Hodgkin lymphoma cell lines (61) but evidence for functional RANK on breast cancer cells is still lacking. Recent abstract data indicates that RANKL induces responses in breast cancer cells. These responses include NF-κB activation, increased mRNA expression of TGF-β and PTHrP, as well as invasion through matrigel (62). These observations are consistent with the presence of functional RANK on breast cancer cells, although this conclusion is based strictly on the apparent lack of alternative signaling pathways for RANKL (9, 20). If breast cancer cells express functional RANK, then it is conceivable that they could proliferate and invade in response to RANKL in the same manner as would mammary epithelial cells during pregnancy. The ability of bone-derived RANKL to promote breast cancer cell proliferation and survival would provide an elegant hypothetical mechanism for breast cancer cell osteotropism. An extension of this hypothesis is the potential for anti-RANKL therapies to have direct anti-tumor effects on breast cancer cells superimposed on their well-established and potent antiresorptive effects. Clearly there are substantial gaps in the body of data that would support this hypothesis of osteotropism, but unfortunately there is also a paucity of internally consistent and testable alternative hypotheses.

3.3 Prostate Cancer

Bone metastases from prostate cancer are typically blastic in nature, so it is not immediately intuitive that OPG/RANK/RANKL would have a significant role in this process. However, most bone metastases from prostate cancer also include an osteolytic component (63-66) and prostate cancer patients with bone metastases frequently have elevated serum markers of bone resorption (67). The stimulus for this osteolytic component is not well understood, and it may merely represent a normal coupling phenomenon that follows prostate cancer stimulation of osteoblasts (68). Recent data suggest that prostate cancer cells may also play a more direct role in stimulating osteoclasts. A bone-metastasizing human prostate cancer cell line (C4-2B) secretes a soluble form of RANKL that directly promotes osteoclastogenesis (Figure 2), an effect which is blocked by OPG (16). Primary human prostate cancer cells have also been shown to express RANKL mRNA, and this expression was apparently upregulated in bone metastases (69). The significance of these observations and their influence on bone resorption are difficult to determine, as OPG mRNA was also elevated in prostate bone metastases (69).

increased osteoclast numbers when injected into the femurs of op/op mice, and OPG treatment reduced osteoclast numbers and skeletal tumor burden by over 90% (106). In these two models, OPG had no effect on tumor burden in non-osseous sites, suggesting that the anti-tumor effects observed in bone were mediated indirectly via the antiresorptive effect of OPG.

Bone pain from metastasis is a potentially debilitating and much feared consequence of disseminated disease. The pathways leading to pain are poorly understood, but recent animal data has provided novel insights that implicate osteoclast activity in this process. The injection osteolytic sarcoma cells into mouse femurs caused extensive bone destruction, bone pain, and pain-related changes in the neurochemical organization of the spinal cord. OPG treatment eliminated osteoclasts and prevented osteolysis, while also inhibiting the pain and pain-related neurochemical changes (107, 108). This study supports a role for osteoclast activity and/or bone resorption in the pathogenesis of bone pain. These data are the first to demonstrate that an antiresorptive agent can reverse the neurochemical changes associated with pain.

It is noteworthy that despite these pharmacologic benefits, OPG did not significantly reduce skeletal tumor burden in this model (107). This finding may be related to the type of tumor used and the route of administration. These tumor cells were directly inoculated into the femur, so it cannot be concluded that these tumor cells were in any way dependent on the bone microenvironment for their growth and/or survival. The lack of tumor burden suppression with OPG treatment could merely reflect the autonomous nature of these tumor cells in bone. In other words, not all osteolytic tumors depend on osteolysis for their growth or survival. For example, osteolytic Walker 256 carcinoma cells metastasize spontaneously to bone and cause extensive osteolysis (109). While the bisphosphonate pamidronate effectively blocked this osteolysis, skeletal tumor burden and tumor cell proliferation actually increased (110). Tumor inoculation into the heart or systemic circulation results in a more stochastic metastatic process, and bone metastases under these conditions are likely to be more dependent on the bone microenvironment. Whenever these routes of inoculation are used for osteolytic tumors, RANKL antagonism has consistently resulted in a decrease in skeletal tumor burden (23, 81, 99). It will be important to challenge these findings by testing a variety of RANKL antagonists in an expanded panel of metastatic tumor models. Head to head comparisons with other classes of antiresorptives will also be helpful to determine whether different mechanisms of antiresorptive action have differential effects on osteoclasts and on tumor burden.

5. CONCLUSIONS

Tumor-induced osteolysis is the major cause of morbidity in patients with bone metastases. Pain, hypercalcemia and pathologic fractures are common features of metastatic bone disease that could be adequately controlled with effective antiresorptive agents. The discovery of OPG/RANK/RANKL has provided a novel set of tools for studying the pathophysiological mechanisms responsible for osteoclast activation. Data reported so far indicates that RANKL is ultimately responsible for the bone resorption induced by virtually all tumors types. OPG, whether from endogenous sources or from pharmacologic administration, neutralizes RANKL and prevents it activating RANK on osteoclasts. Tumor cells have adopted several mechanisms for inducing bone resorption, and most of these mechanisms lead to an excess of RANKL relative to OPG. Tumor cells may produce their own RANKL, but it is more common for tumor cells to secrete factors that induce RANKL expression by host cells such as osteoblasts, stromal cells or T-cells. Tumor cells can also promote bone resorption by causing the suppression of OPG production by host cells. Multiple myeloma cells may also have the unique ability to directly bind and sequester OPG, thereby preventing it from neutralizing RANKL. In limited studies with cancer patients, OPG treatment causes rapid, significant and sustained reductions in markers of bone resorption. In animal models of experimental bone metastasis, OPG and other RANKL antagonists consistently reduce osteoclast numbers and prevent osteolysis. Protection of bone in these models is frequently associated with significant reductions in skeletal tumor burden. These observations provide a compelling rationale for testing the efficacy of RANKL antagonists in patients with bone metastasis.

LIST OF ABBREVIATIONS:

OPG: Osteoprotegerin
RANK: Receptor Activator of Nuclear Factor Kappa B
RANKL: Receptor Activator of Nuclear Factor Kappa B Ligand
TNF-α: Tumor Necrosis Factor Alpha
TR1: TNF Receptor Superfamily Member 1
FDCR-1: Follicular Dendritic Cell Receptor-1
OCIF: Osteoclast Inhibitory Factor
KO: Knockout
OPGL: Osteoprotegerin Ligand
TRANCE: TNF-Related Activation-Induced Cytokine
ODF: Osteoclast Differentiation Factor

72. Penno H, Silfversward CJ, Frost A, Brandstrom H, Nilsson O, Ljunggren O. Osteoprotegerin secretion from prostate cancer is stimulated by cytokines, in vitro. Biochem Biophys Res Comm, 293: 451-455, 2002.
73. Goldring SR, Roelke MS, Petrison KK, Bhan AK. Human giant cell tumors of bone: Identification and characterization of cell types. J Clin Invest, 79: 483-491, 1987.
74. Atkins GJ, Bouralexis S, Haynes DR, Graves SE, Geary SM, Evdokiou A, Zannettino A, Hay S, Findlay DM. Osteoprotegerin inhibits osteoclast formation and bone resorbing activity in giant cell tumors of bone. Bone, 28: 370-377, 2001.
75. Roux S, Amazit L, Meduri G, Guiochon-Mantel A, Milgrom E, Mariette X. RANK (receptor activator of nuclear factor kappa B) and RANK ligand are expressed in giant cell tumors of bone. Am J Clin Pathol, 117: 210-216, 2002.
76. Huang L, Xu J, Wood DJ, Zheng MH. Gene expression of osteoprotegerin ligand, osteoprotegerin, and receptor activator of NF-kB in giant cell tumor of bone. Am J Clin Pathol, 156: 761-767, 2000.
77. Atkins GJ, Haynes DR, Graves SE, Evdokiou A, Hay S, Bouralexis S, Findlay DM. Expression of osteoclast differentiation signals by stromal elements of giant cell tumors. J Bone Min Res, 15: 640-649, 2000.
78. Michigami T, Ihara-Watanabe M, Yamazaki M, Ozono K. Receptor activator of nuclear factor kB ligand (RANKL) is a key molecule of osteoclast formation for bone metastasis in a newly developed model of human neuroblastoma. Cancer Res, 61: 1637-1644, 2001.
79. Nosaka K, Miyamoto T, Sakai T, Mitsuya H, Suda T, Matsuoka M. Mechanisms of hypercalcemia in adult T-cell leukemia: overexpression of receptor activator of nuclear factor kB ligand on adult T-cell leukemia cells. Blood, 99: 634-640, 2002.
80. Sasaki A, Boyce BF, Story B, Wright KR, Chapman M, Boyce R, Mundy GR, Yoneda T. Bisphosphonate risedronate reduces metastatic human breast cancer burden in bone in nude mice. Cancer Res, 55: 3551-3557, 1995.
81. Morony S, Capparelli C, Sarosi I, Lacey DL, Dunstan CR, Kostenuik PJ. Osteoprotegerin inhibits osteolysis and decreases skeletal tumor burden in syngeneic and nude mouse models of experimental bone metastasis. Cancer Res, 61: 4432-4436, 2001.
82. Kostenuik PJ, Singh G, Suyama KL, Orr FW. Stimulation of bone resorption results in a selective increase in the growth rate of spontaneously metastatic Walker 256 cancer cells in bone. Clin Exp Metastasis, 10: 411-418, 1992.
83. Paget S. The distribution of secondary growths in cancer of the breast. Lancet, 1: 571-573, 1889.
84. Berrettoni BA, Carter JR. Mechanisms of Cancer Metastasis to Bone. J Bone Joint Surg, 68-A: 308-312, 1986.
85. Akatsu T, Murakami T, Ono K, Nishikawa M, Tsuda E, Mochizuki SI, Fujise N, Higashio K, Motoyoshi K, Yamamoto M, Nagata N. Osteoclastogenesis inhibitory factor exhibits hypocalcemic effects in normal mice and in hypercalcemic nude mice carrying tumors associated with humoral hypercalcemia of malignancy. Bone, 23: 495-498, 1998.
86. Hakeda Y, Kobayashi Y, Yamaguchi K, Yasuda H, Tsuda E, Higashio K, Miyata T, Kumegawa M. Osteoclastogenesis inhibitory factor (OCIF) directly inhibits bone-

resorbing activity of isolated mature osteoclasts. Biochem Biophys Res Comm, 251: 796-801, 1998.

87. Yamamoto M, Murakami T, Nishikawa M, Tsuda E, Mochizuki SI, Higashio K, Akatsu T, Motoyoshi K, Nagata N. Hypocalcemic effect of osteoclastogenesis inhibitory factor/osteoprotegerin in the thyroparathyroidectomized rat. Endocrinol, 139: 4012-4015, 1998.
88. Capparelli C, Kostenuik PJ, Morony S, Starnes C, Weimann B, Van G, Scully S, Qi M, Lacey DL, Dunstan CR. Osteoprotegerin prevents and reverses hypercalcemia in a murine model of humoral hypercalcemia of malignancy. Cancer Res, 60: 783-787, 2000.
89. Martin TJ. Humoral Hypercalcemia of Malignancy. Bone Min, 4: 83-89, 1988.
90. Shipley PJ, Shevrin DH, Kukreja SC. Increased Renal Calcium Reabsorption in an Animal Model of Hypercalcemia of Human Malignancy. J Bone Min Res, 3: 555-560, 1988.
91. Thiebaud D, Jaeger P, Burckhardt P. Response to retreatment of malignant hypercalcemia with the bisphosphonate AHPrBP (APD): Respective role of kidney and bone. J Bone Min Res, 5: 221-226, 1990.
92. Kostenuik PJ, Morony S, Capparelli C, Lacey DL, Dunstan C. Comparison of the inhibitory effects of osteoprotegerin and of APD on PTHrP-mediated hypercalcemia and bone remodeling. (Abst) J Bone Min Res, 14(Suppl 1), S166. 1999.
93. Capparelli C, Kostenuik, PJ, Morony S, Starnes C, Weimann B, Sarosi I, Lacey DL, Dunstan C. Comparison of osteoprotegerin and pamidronate in a murine model of humoral hypercalcemia of malignancy. (Abst) J Bone Min Res. 14(Suppl 1): S163, 1999.
94. Caligaris-Cappio F, Bergui L, Gregoretti MG, Gaidano G, Gaboli M, Schena M, Zambonin-Zallone AZ, Marchiso PC. Role of bone marrow stromal cells in the growth of human multiple myeloma. Blood, 77: 2688-2693, 1991.
95. Vanderkerken K, De Leenheer E, Shipman C, Asosingh K, Willems A, van Camp B, Croucher P. Recombinant osteoprotegerin decreases tumor burden and increases survival in a murine model of multiple myeloma. Cancer Res, 63: 287-289, 2003.
96. Mansi JL, Berger U, McDonnell T, Pople A, Rayter Z, Gazet JC, Coombes RC. The fate of bone marrow micrometastases in patients with primary breast cancer. J Clin Oncol, 7: 445-449, 1989.
97. Yamashita K, Ueda T, Komatsubara Y, Koyama H, Inaji H, Yonenobu K, Ono K. Breast cancer with bone-only metastases. Cancer, 68: 634-637, 1991.
98. Chukwuma Chiedozi L. Prognostic significance of exclusive skeletal metastases in stage IV primary carcinoma of the breast. Surg Gynecol Obst, 167: 303-306, 1988.
99. Morony S, Warmington K, Tan H, Shalhoub V, Chow JWM, Dunstan CR, Lacey DL, Kostenuik, PJ. OPG inhibits the progression of bone destruction and skeletal tumor burden in mice with established osteolytic MDA-231 breast cancer metastases. (Abst) J Bone Min Res, 17(Suppl 1): S147, 2002.
100. Kiefer JA, Vessella RL, Quinn JE, Odman A, Zhang J, Keller ET, Corey E. The effect of osteoprotegerin administration on the intra-tibial growth of the osteoblastic LuCaP 23.1 prostate cancer zenograft. (Abst) J Bone Min Res, 17(Suppl 1): S230, 2002.

101. Chakal-Roy M, Niemeyer C, Moore MA, Zetter BR. Stimulation of human prostatic carcinoma cell growth by factors present in human bone marrow. J Clin Invest, 84: 43-50, 1989.
102. Polychronakos C, Janthly U, Lehoux JG, Koutsilieris M. Mitogenic effects of insulin and insulin-like growth factors on PA-III rat prostate adenocarcinoma cells: Characterization of the receptors involved. Prostate, 19: 313-321, 1991.
103. Ritchie CK, Andrews LR, Thomas KG, Tindall DJ, Fitzpatrick LA. The effects of growth factors associated with osteoblasts on prostate carcinoma proliferation and chemotaxis: Implications for the development of metastatic disease. Endocrinol, 138: 1145-1150, 1997.
104. Lamm M, Sintich SM, Lee C. A proliferative effect of transforming growth factor-b1 on a human prostate cancer cell line, TSU-Pr1. Endocrinol, 139: 787-790, 1998.
105. Rubin J, Chung L, Fan X, Zhu L, Murphy TC, Nanes MS, Rosen CJ. Bone microenvironment triggers IGF-1 release from prostate carcinoma. (Abst) J Bone Min Res, 17(Suppl 1): S148, 2002.
106. Clohisy DR, Ramnaraine ML, Scully S, Qi M, Van G, Tan HL, Lacey DL. Osteoprotegerin inhibits tumor-induced osteoclastogenesis and bone tumor growth in osteopetrotic mice. J Orthopaedic Res, 18: 967-976, 2000.
107. Honore P, Luger NM, Sabino M, Schwei MJ, Rogers SD, Mach DB, O'Keefe PF, Ramnaraine ML, Clohisy DR, Mantyh PW. Osteoprotegerin blocks bone cancer-induced skeletal destruction, skeletal pain and pain-related neurochemical reorganization of the spinal cord. Nature Med, 6: 521-528, 2000.
108. Luger NM, Honore P, Sabino M, Schwei MJ, Rogers SD, Mach DB, Clohisy DR, Mantyh PW. Osteoprotegerin diminishes advanced cancer pain. Cancer Res, 61: 4038-4047, 2001.
109. Kostenuik PJ, Singh G., Suyama KL, Orr FW. A quantitative model for spontaneous bone metastasis: Evidence for a mitogenic effect of bone on Walker 256 cancer cells. Clin Exp Metastasis, 10: 403-410, 1992.
110. Kostenuik PJ, Orr FW, Suyama KL, Singh G. Increased growth rate and tumor burden of spontaneously metastatic Walker 256 cancer cells in the skeleton of bisphosphonate-treated rats. Cancer Res, 53: 5452-5457, 1993.

Chapter 12

ROLE OF MATRIX METALLOPROTEINASES IN BONE METASTASIS FROM HUMAN BREAST AND PROSTATE CANCER

Wilhelmina C.M. Duivenvoorden* and Gurmit Singh
Juravinski Cancer Centre, McMaster University, Hamilton Ontario, Canada
**Current address: Northwestern Ontario Regional Cancer Centre, Thunder Bay Ontario, Canada*

1. INCIDENCE AND MANIFESTATION OF BONE METASTASIS

Bone metastases are a significant problem in patients with cancer of the breast and prostate. Bone metastases are associated with extensive morbidity and mortality. They cause clinical disease due to extensive, intractable bone pain, pathological fractures, and spinal cord compression and leads eventually to death. 70% of patients that die of breast cancer have noticeable disease in their bones (1, 2). Similar numbers are found for prostate cancer patients (2). Bone disease is also a major problem in multiple myeloma patients. The manifestation of the bone involvement is distinct for the three types of cancers.

Bone metastasis from breast carcinoma is frequently associated with osteolysis leading to extensive morbidity from bone pain, fractures and hypercalcaemia (3). Data from the MD Anderson Cancer Centre show that out of the 1171 patients that were entered on treatment for metastatic breast cancer, two thirds had involvement of bone. 180 of these patients had metastasis in bone only, of those 48% had osteolytic disease, 13% pure osteoblastic and the remaining presented with mixed metastasis. The most common skeletal areas involved are the pelvis and lumbosacral spine (4).

G. Singh and W. Orr (eds.), Bone Metastasis and Molecular Mechanisms, 241-276.

Biochemical markers for bone metastasis in breast cancer patients are increased serum alkaline phosphatase, a marker of bone deposition, and urinary galactosyl-hydroxylysine, a marker of collagen catabolism (5). Tumor-associated hypercalcaemia is observed in 30% of breast cancer patients with bone involvement (6).

Prostate cancer patients exhibit primarily osteoblastic or osteosclerotic bone disease. The presence of tumor cells in the bone causes stimulation of osteoblastic activity resulting in increased bone mass adjacent to the tumor cells (7). However, increased bone resorption has also been documented histologically and biochemically in prostate cancer patients (8). Metabolic changes that are associated with bone metastasis in prostate cancer are hypocalcaemia and increased serum bone alkaline phosphatase as a marker of osteoblastic activity. More surprisingly, increased urinary deoxypyridoline and pyridinoline cross-linked carboxyterminal telopeptide of type I collagen, which are both markers of osteoclastic activity, have been observed in prostate cancer patients with metastatic bone disease (9).

Multiple myeloma is a malignant neoplasm resulting from monoclonal proliferation of plasma cells, which is associated with the overproduction of monoclonal IgG, IgA and/or light chains. The clinical presentation of the disease is often characterized by bone pain as a result of very extensive bone destruction. As a consequence of the myeloma cell infiltration an increase in osteoclastic activity and proliferation occurs mediated by the release of osteoclast-activating factors produced locally in the bone microenvironment by cells of both tumor and non-tumor origin (10). In about 30% of all multiple myeloma patients tumor-associated hypercalcaemia is observed (6).

2. MATRIX METALLOPROTEINASES

Matrix metalloproteinases (MMPs) are a large class of closely related collagenases involved in degradation and remodelling of the extracellular matrix in embryogenesis and tissue repair [recently reviewed in (11, 12)]. The activity of MMPs is tightly regulated in physiological situations where extracellular remodelling must occur, e.g., in morphogenesis and wound healing. The enzymes can be divided into six broad classes on the basis of sequence homology and substrate specificity (Table 1). Collectively, MMPs are capable of degrading all of the components of the extracellular matrix (13, 14). One class of MMPs consists of the membrane-bound MMPs. MT1-MMP, MT2-MMP, MT3-MMP and MT5-MMP all contain a transmembrane domain, which facilitates the cell-mediated activation of 72-kDa type IV collagenase (MMP-2) (15-20), whereas MT4-MMP and MT6-MMP are attached to the membrane through a glycosylphosphatidylinositol (GPI)-

anchor. The more recently discovered MMP-23 contains a cysteine array and a unique interleukin-1 receptor-related domain (21). It is a type II transmembrane MMP with an N-terminal signal anchor (22).

Table 1. Human family of matrix metalloproteinases and their classical substrates

Class of MMPs	MMP	Substrate
Interstitial collagenases	Interstitial collagenase (MMP-1) Neutrophil collagenase (MMP-8) Collagenase-3 (MMP-13)	Type I, II, and III fibrillar collagens
Stromelysins	Stromelysin-1 (MMP-3) Stromelysin-2 (MMP-10)	Proteoglycans, laminin, type IV collagen and type X collagen
Matrilysins	Matrilysin (MMP-7)	Fibronectin, laminin, type IV and X collagen
	Matrilysin-2 (MMP-26)	-
Type IV collagenases	72-kDa type IV collagenase (MMP-2) 92-kDa type IV collagenase (MMP-9)	Type IV and type V non-fibrillar collagens, type VII collagen, fibronectin, type X collagen, elastin
Furin-activatable MMPs	Stromelysin-3 (MMP-11)	α1-proteinase inhibitor
	Epilysin (MMP-28)	Casein
Membrane type MMPs	MT1-MMP (MMP-14) MT2-MMP (MMP-15) MT3-MMP (MMP-16)	Latent MMP-2
	MT4-MMP (MMP-17)	-
	MT5-MMP (MMP-24)	Latent MMP-2
	MT6-MMP (MMP-25, Leukolysin)	Collagen IV
Type II transmembrane MMPs	MMP-23	
Other MMPs	Metalloelastase (MMP-12)	Elastin, type IV collagen, laminin, fibronectin
	MMP-19	Type IV collagen, laminin, fibronectin, aggrecan
	Enamelysin (MMP-20)	Amelogenin, type XVIII collagen
	MMP-27	-

2.1 Regulation of MMP Expression and Activity

Matrix metalloproteinase activity is tightly regulated and occurs at different levels. Regulation of gene expression occurs at both the transcriptional and posttranscriptional level. AP-1 and ETS binding sites are among the most important *cis*-acting elements found in the promoter regions of the majority of the MMP genes, except for MMP-2. They are involved in the stimulation of MMP gene expression by phorbol esters, serum, and IL-1 (23, 24). Epidermal growth factor (EGF) has been shown to increase the transcription of interstitial collagenase (MMP-1) in human breast adenocarcinoma MDA-MB-231 cells (25). Transforming growth factor-β1 (TGF-β1) and retinoic acid inhibit the expression of MMP-1 at the transcriptional level (26-28). In the repression by TGF-β1, the AP-1 site cooperates with the TIE (transforming growth factor inhibitor element) site (29), whereas more distal sites of the promoter of MMP-1 are involved in the repression by all-*trans*-retinoic acid (27).

MMPs are secreted as latent enzymes that have to be proteolytically modified for activation. They are activated by removal of a portion of the amino-terminal part of the enzyme (30). *In vivo* activation occurs through a cascade of activation of various latent proteinases. Serine proteases such as trypsin can activate various latent MMPs. Another serine protease, plasmin, can be both directly involved in the degradation of collagen I as well as activate latent MMP-1 and stromelysin-1 (MMP-3) (31). Plasmin in turn is generated from plasminogen through the action of predominantly the urokinase-type plasminogen activator cascade (32). Some members of the MMP family can directly activate other MMPs. For example, collagenase-3 (MMP-13) can be activated by MT1-MMP, MMP-3 and MMP-2 (33, 34). MMP-3 can carry out the final activation step of MMP-1 and MMP-3 after they have been cleaved by plasmin or trypsin. MMP-3 can also completely activate latent 92-kDa type IV collagenase (MMP-9) (35).

MMP-2 is in several regards distinct from the other members of the MMP family. Firstly, it is not activated in a similar fashion as the other MMPs. MMP-2 cannot be activated by plasmin, trypsin, chymotrypsin, thrombin, cathepsin G or MMP-3 (36), but is activated through a mechanism involving membrane-bound proteins. As recently as 1991 Ward *et al.* reported the activation of latent MMP-2 by plasma membranes isolated from fibroblasts (37). Using degenerate primers homologous to the conserved sequences in the cysteine switch region and the catalytic domain of MMPs led to the cloning of the first membrane-type MMP, MT1-MMP. Expression of this protein in COS-1 cells shows its presence on the cell surface (38).

Tissue inhibitors of metalloproteinases (TIMPs) are the natural endogenous inhibitors of MMPs. TIMPs are small proteins that non-covalently form 1:1 complexes with specific MMPs, blocking their proteolytic effect (39). TIMP-1 specifically binds to most MMP family members, whereas TIMP-2 binds and inhibits MMP-2. This can occur through two distinct mechanisms; binding to proMMP-2 and thereby inhibiting the cleavage into active MMP-2 or by binding to MMP-2 and inhibiting its activity (37). TIMP-3 is associated with the extracellular matrix and not soluble like the other three TIMPs (40). The latest member of the TIMP family, TIMP-4, was cloned in 1996 from a heart cDNA library (42). TIMP-3 and TIMP-1 are equally effective in inhibiting MMP-1, MMP-2, MMP-3 and 92-kDa type IV collagenase (MMP-9) (41). A balance between MMPs and TIMPs determines the overall collagenolytic activity.

Unlike other MMPs, MMP-2 is usually found complexed with TIMP-2 through their respective C-terminal domains. A second binding site for TIMP-2 on the N-terminal part of the MMP-2 distinct from the active site also exists (43). Ultimately the balance of TIMP-2 over MMP-2 will decide whether MMP-2 is activated by MT1-MMP. TIMP-2 actually has a dual effect on the activation of proMMP-2; at low concentrations TIMP-2 enhances MMP-2 activation, whereas at high concentrations it acts inhibitory. When the ratio of TIMP-2:MMP-2 is between 1 and 2, TIMP-2 through its N-terminal domain binds to MT1-MMP and through its C-terminal end binds to the C-terminal domain of proMMP-2, which can subsequently be presented to and activated by a neighbouring MT1-MMP molecule. The MT1-MMP molecule does not necessarily have to be located on the same cell. If the ratio is greater than 2 there is enough TIMP-2 to bind to proMMP-2 and, separately, to MT1-MMP. This therefore does not lead to activation (44).

Lastly, MMPs are inactivated through degradation. Plasmin, which is involved in the activation of MMPs, can also play, under other circumstances, a role in the degradation process of MMPs (45). In the presence of plasmin, uncomplexed MMP-2 is degraded, whereas the binding of TIMP-2 to MMP-2 prevents the degradation by plasmin (46, 47). Interaction of MMP-2 and MMP-9 with the cell surface may also partially protect the MMPs from degradation (46). MT1-MMP degradation into an inactive 43 kDa form occurs within 1-4 h after translation, which parallels the activation of MMP-2. Interestingly, this process is inhibitable by a synthetic MMP inhibitor (45). Stromelysin-3 (MMP-11) is inactivated in a similar MMP-dependent manner (48).

2.2 Non-Classical MMP Substrates

More recently novel MMP substrates other than components of the extracellular matrix have been discovered. The ability of MMPs to cleave growth factors, proteins involved in cell adhesion, and growth factor receptors suggests different mechanisms of action for MMPs in the development of metastatic cancer.

MMP-2 and MMP-9 can release TGF-β from its latent complex (49). Tumor necrosis factor-α (TNF-α), a potent pro-inflammatory cytokine, is expressed as a 26-kDa precursor found anchored on the membrane of leukocytes. In order for TNF-α to become biologically active it has to be proteolytically cleaved. Synthetic MMP inhibitors have been found to specifically inhibit this process. Matrilysin (MMP-7), stromelysin-1 (MMP-3), MMP-1, and to a slightly lesser extent MMP-2 and MMP-9 are capable of releasing TNF-α (50). Processing of the precursor of IL-1β into its biologically active form can be carried out by MMP-3 and MMP-9 and, to a lesser extent, MMP-2, but not by MMP-1. This process is independent of caspase-1 (IL-1β-converting enzyme) (51).

Proteins involved in cell adhesion, such as CD44, E-cadherin and laminin, are also substrates for MMPs. MT1-MMP has been shown to cleave the ecto-domain of the CD44 receptor (52). CD44 is the main cell surface receptor for hyaluronate, a component of the extracellular matrix. Treatment with 1,10-phenanthroline, a general MMP-inhibitor, prevents cleavage and results in the suppression of lung cancer cell migration on hyaluronate as a substrate (53). Upon cleavage of E-cadherin by MMP-7 and MMP-3, the released E-cadherin fragment can promote invasion (54). Laminin-5 can be cleaved by MMP-2, which results in the exposure of a cryptic site on laminin-5 that induces cell motility (55).

MMPs are involved in the shedding of the HER2/*neu* receptor, the receptor that is frequently overexpressed in human breast cancer. TIMP-1, but not TIMP-2, EDTA and a synthetic MMP inhibitor, batimastat, can inhibit the shedding. Cleavage of the extracellular domain of the HER2/*neu* receptor is associated with poor prognosis and resistance to chemotherapy and endocrine therapy in breast cancer, since this truncated HER2 protein has the capacity to enhance signalling (56). The shedding of the interleukin-6 receptor observed in multiple myeloma can also be inhibited by MMP-inhibitors (TIMP-3 and batimastat, but not TIMP-1 or -2) (57). Similarly, TIMP-3-overexpressing colon carcinoma cells show increased sensitivity towards apoptosis induced by serum starvation or hydrogen peroxide treatment probably through stabilization of TNF-α receptors on the cells' surface (58).

Metalloelastase (MMP-12) cleaves plasminogen to generate angiostatin, a protein with anti-angiogenic properties. In hepatocellular carcinoma patients undergoing curative partial hepatectomy a significant association between MMP-12 mRNA and angiostatin protein is reported with angiostatin found in the tumorous tissue and a correlation with survival (59). Such non-classical properties offer an additional role for MMPs in tumor progression.

2.3 MMP Expression and Activity in Cancer

Matrix metalloproteinases are involved in various steps of the development of metastasis, since they are able to degrade the extracellular matrix and the components of basement membranes, which underlie the endothelial cells. They can thus facilitate access to blood vessels and allow the development of tumor growth at distant sites (31, 60). There is substantial evidence that a positive correlation between the expression of MMPs and the invasiveness and/or grade of the tumor exists. Animal and *in vitro* experiments have provided extensive evidence to support the role of MMPs in the process of invasion and metastasis. A direct correlation between the lung metastatic potential of cancer cells and the capacity to degrade type IV collagen was first reported in 1980 (61). Those initial findings have been confirmed in other experiments using differentially metastatic clones of rat mammary adenocarcinoma cells (62) and cell hybrids made from cells with different metastatic potential (63). In oncogene-transformed rat cell lines with different metastatic properties the levels of the stromelysin-1 and -2 (MMP-3 and MMP-10), correlate positively with the metastatic phenotype of the cells, whereas the expression of MMP-2 and MMP-9 is not associated with metastasis in these cell lines (64). Data from gene-knockout studies in animals underline the importance of the role of MMPs in tumor and metastasis development. A strain of mice prone to develop intestinal adenoma that is also deficient for MMP-7 shows a 58% reduction in the amount of tumors compared to MMP-7 +/+ mice (65). Stromelysin-3 (MMP-11)-deficient mice demonstrate a reduction in DMBA-induced carcinoma incidence and tumor size (66). In MMP-9-deficient mice the number of metastatic colonies from B16/BL6 and Lewis lung carcinoma decreases by 45 and 59% respectively (67).

To date, a correlation between elevated MMP expression and the stage of the disease, diagnosis or survival has been reported for many different types of human cancers. Elevation of MMP-9 has been documented in breast (68), pancreatic (69), prostate (70, 71), ovarian (72, 73), and bladder cancer (74), lung tumors, squamous cell carcinoma of the uterine cervix (75), and also hepatocellular carcinoma (76). Other MMPs have been associated with tumor progression as well. High levels of MMP-1 protein (77) and increased collagenolytic activity have been observed in colorectal cancer (78, 79). MMP-1 has also been found overexpressed in head and neck squamous cell carcinomas. In these cancers this coincided with an overexpression of MMP-10 (80). In human breast adenocarcinomas MMP-1 immunoreactivity correlates inversely with stage and progesterone receptor status of the cancer, however, only when the immunoreactivity found in the stromal cells, but not in cancer cells is considered (81). Another collagenase, collagenase-3 or MMP-13, originally cloned from breast cancer tissue (82) has been localized to tumor cells in squamous cell carcinoma of the head and neck (83) and invasive vulvar squamous cell carcinomas (84). In breast carcinoma, an inverse correlation between MMP-11 and long-term survival has been observed both at the level of mRNA expression (in 55 patients with invasive breast cancer) (85) and the level of protein expression (in 111 patients) (86). MMP-7 expression is confined to samples of prostate cancer tissue, and is hardly detectable in normal or hyperplastic prostate tissue (87). MMP-2 expression has been correlated to invasiveness in ovarian cancer (88, 89).

MMP-2 has been found overexpressed on the mRNA level in pancreatic (69), prostate (90) and colorectal cancer (91). Active MMP-2, but not latent MMP-2, has been found to correlate with invasiveness in bladder cancer (74) and with tumor grade in malignant breast cancer (68). An elevation of MT1-MMP and the association with an increased ratio of active MMP-2 over latent MMP-2 has been reported in several cancers. The expression of MT1-MMP in breast adenocarcinoma correlates with lymph node and distant metastasis and clinical stage of the tumor. This coincides with an increased activation of proMMP-2 into active MMP-2 and correlates with MT1-MMP, but not MT2-MMP or MT3-MMP mRNA expression (92). Similar results were found for papillary thyroid carcinomas (93), gastric carcinoma (94-96), brain tumors, including astrocytomas and glioblastomas (97), and hepatocellular carcinomas (98, 99).

In squamous cell carcinoma of the uterine cervix, the ratio of MMP-2+MMP-9 over TIMP-1+TIMP-2 has been determined. A high ratio of MMP:TIMP is associated with a poor prognosis (100). Similarly, in pancreatic tumors the mRNA of MMP-2 and MMP-9 is elevated compared to control tissue, and the cancerous tissue shows a concomitant increase in the levels of TIMP-1 and TIMP-2 (69). No ratio was determined in this study. Many of these data are derived from studies using *in situ* hybridization or RT-PCR, which can only detect quantity and location of the transcript or Northern blotting which can only be employed semi-quantitatively. Immunohistochemistry, which has also been widely used, localizes specific proteins, but is limited through the sensitivity and specificity of the antibodies used. A true measure that takes into account the amount of active protein, the availability, and binding to TIMPs, is *in situ* enzymography. However, this technique is limited to only a few substrates (gelatin, casein) and will not distinguish between different MMPs that cleave the same substrate. It has been employed in an elegant study looking at human papillary thyroid carcinoma. The authors performed a thorough study to establish a relationship between MT1-MMP expression and active MMP-2. Normal control, follicular adenoma and carcinoma tissue homogenates were used for ELISA, gelatin enzymography and Northern blot analysis for MT1-MMPs and showed a strong correlation between the stage of the disease and the level of activation of MMP-2. Levels of MT1-MMP as determined by Northern blot correlated with the activation of MMP-2 and also with lymph node metastases. *In situ* hybridization and immunohistochemistry showed that MT1-MMP, MT2-MMP and MMP-2 are expressed by both tumor and stromal cells, however, *in situ* enzymography revealed that the activity is predominantly present in the carcinoma cells (93).

2.4 TIMP Expression in Cancer

As stated before, the overall collagenolytic activity of cancer cells is determined by a balance between active enzymes and TIMPs. Classical experimental studies have reported that overexpression or addition of recombinant TIMP in metastatic cells is associated with an inhibition of invasive and metastatic potential *in vitro* and *in vivo* (101-104) and neovascularization can be blocked (105). TIMP-1, -2 or -3 gene delivery using adenovirus techniques in two metastatic melanoma cell lines can inhibit invasion through a reconstituted basement membrane with TIMP-3 overexpression being the most effective (106). TIMP-3- or TIMP-4-transfected human mammary adenocarcinoma MDA-MB-435 cells show significantly slower tumor growth *in vivo* compared to control cells (107, 108). Injection of TIMP-2-transfected breast cancer MDA-MB-231 cells into nude mice results in significantly less radiologically detectable osteolytic bone tumors and coincides with an increased survival of the mice (109). When taking into consideration both MMPs and TIMPs, highly metastatic clones of human prostate cancer PC-3 cells have been found to contain relatively high levels of MMP-2 and low amounts of TIMP-2 when compared to the less invasive clones (110). Reduced levels of free TIMP are associated with higher levels of active MMP-2 in malignant explant prostate cultures when compared to normal and benign prostate samples (111). Samples obtained from gastric cancer patients dying from the disease are more likely to have a lower percentage of TIMP-2 expressing cells and high levels of MMP-2 expressing cells (112). Immunolabelling of gastric cancer tissue revealed a correlation between TIMP-2 staining and metastasis. Among advanced gastric carcinomas cases neoplasms with diffuse and strong staining for TIMP-2 have less frequently nodal metastasis (29%) when compared to the neoplasms that show focal and weak TIMP-2 staining (69% of these cases have metastasis) (113). A comparison of cutaneous basal and squamous cell carcinoma revealed significantly higher levels of TIMP-2 mRNA in the cutaneous basal carcinoma tissue samples, suggesting osteoclastic bone degradation is more prominent, while in the later stages of bone destruction the tumor cells seem to mediate the bone resorption. At the later stages the osteoclasts are absent. Human tumor samples from various malignant diseases similarly show these two distinct phases of bone resorption (132). Tumor-associated macrophages isolated from breast cancer tissue have the potential to differentiate into TRAP (tartrate-resistant acid phosphatase)-positive multinucleated cells when co-cultured with osteoblast-like cells (133). These osteoclast-like multinucleated cells can resorb bone, however without the presence of the ruffled border structure that is characteristic for osteoclasts (130). It has been previously shown in our laboratory that bone metastatic cancer cells such as human prostate adenocarcinoma PC-3 cells can directly degrade osteoid-like extracellular matrices and fetal rat calvarial bone *in vitro* and that MMPs are involved in the process (134). All these tumor and tumor-associated cell types possess the potential to degrade collagenous matrix and thereby expose bone mineral, which may stimulate osteoclastic bone resorption.

3.1 MMP Expression in Bone and Bone Metastasis

In addition to cysteine proteinases, especially cathepsin K (135, 136), MMPs are believed to contribute to the physiological bone matrix degradation. MMP-1 is the most important among the MMP family members, since it specifically degrades native type I collagen, the protein most abundantly present in the organic matrix of the bone. More recently another interstitial collagenase, MMP-13, has been found to be able to degrade native type I collagen. However, the role of MMP-13 appears less significant in bone resorption, since it more efficiently degrades type II collagen. MMP-13 can be immunolocalized in prepubertal bone to osteoblasts only, and is absent from the epiphyseal area of adult bone. MMP-13 might therefore be more important during primary and secondary epiphyseal ossification (137). MMP-2, although to a lesser extent, is also able to degrade native type I collagen (31), whereas MMP-2 and MMP-9 (138, 139) are known to attack degraded type I collagen.

MMP-1, MMP-2, MMP-9 and both TIMP-1 and -2 have been identified in cultured human osteoblasts (140). In human bone tissue samples MMP-1 has been immunolocalized to both the lining osteoblasts and the cells synthesizing matrix (141). Immunohistochemistry experiments also show that MMP-1 is present in osteoblasts to a much higher extent than in the osteoclasts. This lends support to the hypothesis that osteoblast-derived MMPs play a role in the removal of surface collagenous osteoid, which precedes the osteoclast attachment and the actual bone resorption. *In situ* hybridization, using antisense MMP-9, shows that MMP-9 localizes to the osteoclasts, whereas osteoblasts show only very little MMP-9 staining and not in all cases (142). The MMPs secreted by the osteoclast, the only cell in the bone with the definitive ability to degrade mineralized matrix, are unlikely to be involved in the initial stages of resorption in which bone mineral is dissolved in a highly acidic environment. However, at a later stage when the subcellular zone approaches neutral pH, MMPs may be secreted by the osteoclasts in order to degrade unmineralized matrix.

In an elaborate immunohistochemical study we compared the expression of MMP-1, MMP-2, MMP-9, MT1 MMP and TIMP-1 and TIMP-2 in 31 archival cases of bone metastasis from breast carcinoma to the expression in specimens of primary breast cancer, lymph nodes (from breast cancer patients), and normal breast (143). In tumor-associated fibroblasts TIMP-1 expression is increased in bone metastasis specimens when compared with primary and lymph node tumors. For the MMPs, no major differences between bone metastases and primary or lymph node tumors are found. MMP-1, MT1-MMP and TIMP-1 staining is observed in tumor cells, while MMP-1, MMP-2 and TIMP-2 staining is typically seen in fibroblasts associated with the tumor. The expression of both MMP-2 and MMP-9 is markedly increased in desmoplastic fibroblasts in primary and metastatic tumors as compared to fibroblasts in normal breast tissue. The expression and localization of MMP-1, MMP-9 and TIMP-1 in bone cells in metastatic bone corresponds to what has been described in normal bone suggesting that the expression of these enzymes is not affected by the presence of tumor. However, and not surprisingly, the number and activity of both osteoblasts and osteoclasts is greatly increased in bone metastatic samples (143).

3.2 Expression of MMPs as a Result of Tumor Cell-Invasion

Studies have shown that the stromal expression of numerous MMPs is frequently more prominent than expression by tumor cells themselves. In addition the pattern of MMP expression is tissue-specific. In breast cancer, where many different members of the MMP family are expressed, MMP-1, MMP-3, MT1-MMP and MMP-2 are found in the stromal cells at the mRNA level (81, 144-149). In contrast, by immunohistochemistry MMP-1 and MMP-3 protein are detected predominantly in cancer cells, and only in some cases in stromal cells (81). MMP-2 protein is also found localized in tumor cells (148, 150, 151). Similarly, MT1-MMP protein is localized to the tumor cells in one study (92), but to tumor cells and stromal cells in another (146). MMP-11 has been localized to the stromal cells both by *in situ* hybridization and immunohistochemistry (85, 86, 152). MMP-13, on the mRNA and protein level, is confined to the tumor cells (82). MMP-9 has been demonstrated to localize to macrophages, smooth muscle cells and neutrophils (153). In other studies MMP-9 has been localized to tumor cells, both by *in situ* hybridization (68) and immunohistochemically (151). Immunohistochemical localization of MMPs has been problematic. Some studies localize a certain MMP to fibroblasts, while others describe the same MMP localized to tumor cells, depending on the antibody used. In addition, the results sometimes contradict the findings of *in situ* hybridization experiments.

Other cancers that are associated with bone metastases have been less extensively studied. In prostate carcinoma tissue MMP-2 is expressed by the epithelial neoplastic cells (70, 90, 154) with very little MMP-2 immunostaining in the stromal cells, and only in prostate adenocarcinoma and not in hyperplastic or normal prostate tissue (70). Immunohistochemistry has demonstrated MMP-9 antigenicity in both stromal and epithelial structures of the majority of prostate carcinoma specimens (155). *In situ* hybridization of prostate cancer tissue shows expression of MMP-7 in epithelial cells only and not in the stroma (87). In multiple myeloma the presence of the malignant cells in the bone has a very profound effect on the host tissue. MMP-2 and MMP-9 activity is found in the myeloma cells, whereas the myeloma cells induce MMP-1 expression in the bone marrow stromal cells. MMP-2 activity contributed by the stromal cells is activated in the presence of myeloma cells (156). The tissue- and cell-specific expression of MMPs might contribute to the different characteristics of bone metastasis from various types of primary cancers.

The spread of breast tumor cells to bone is typically accompanied by extensive osteolysis of mineralized collagenous bone matrix. Human breast cancer cells injected into the femora of mice induce an increase in osteoclast number at sites of tumor osteolysis. Conditioned medium derived from the cancer cells has an analogous effect *in vitro* (157, 158). In prostate cancer the presence of tumor cells in the bone stimulates osteoblastic activity resulting in increased bone mass adjacent to the tumor cells. Reciprocal interactions between prostate cancer cells and bone stroma appear to account for the typical osteoblastic response (159-161).

Degradation of collagenous bone matrix in bone metastasis may be the result of increased MMP expression that can occur via several different mechanisms. Tumor cells themselves secrete MMPs (162, 163) that are potentially upregulated during metastasis. Tumor cells also produce cytokines and growth factors that can affect the MMP expression in stromal cells. Conditioned medium derived from human breast adenocarcinoma H-31 cells stimulates the degradation of type I collagen by mouse osteoblast-like cells and bone resorption *in vitro* (164). Human breast cancer cells express and produce interleukin-6 as well as interleukin-11, both potent stimulators of osteoclast development (165). Other factors that could be specifically involved in the upregulation of MMP mRNA expression are interleukin-1 and TNF-α (24, 156). Endothelial cell monolayers have been shown to become increasingly permeable when incubated with cancer cell-conditioned media, an effect inhibitable by 1,10-phenanthroline (166).

Membrane-bound proteins, such as EMMPRIN (Extracellular Matrix MetalloProteinase Inducer), are also involved in the induction of MMP expression in stromal cells. EMMPRIN is highly enriched around the cell's surface and present in tumor cells of lung and breast cancer, but not in normal tissue surrounding the tumor or non-cancerous tissue (167). EMMPRIN isolated from lung carcinoma LX-1 cells has been shown to stimulate production of MMP-1 in fibroblasts (168).

We applied an *in vitro* model system to study the effect of bone-metastatic tumor cells on MMP expression in different human cell lines representative of cell populations present in the bone. We used two types of co-culture systems with the following human cell lines, (i) osteoblast-like cells Saos-2 (169), (ii) GCT, a cell line of monocytic origin (170) with many properties of osteoclasts including TRAP-activity and CD68 antigen expression, (iii) HUV-EC-C, primary endothelial cells derived from a umbilical cord vein (171), and (iv) fibroblast cells (Hf-172). Firstly, we used a co-culture consisting of a monolayer of bone-type cells with human bone-metastatic cancer cells (human mammary adenocarcinoma MDA-MB-231 or human prostate adenocarcinoma PC-3 cells) seeded onto the first monolayer. The second culture system consisted of conditioned medium collected from MDA-MB-231 or PC-3 cells, which was then added to the serum-free medium of cells representative of bone for 24 h.

Our results, shown in Figures 1 A-E, demonstrate that the presence of tumor cells causes the most dramatic results in endothelial cells, but an increase in MMP-1 protein is also observed in all other cells used. The addition of cancer cell-conditioned media only significantly increases MMP-1 protein in fibroblasts. In bone metastasis the presence of tumor cells can thus have an indirect stimulating effect on the expression of MMP-1, one of the major enzymes responsible for the initial degradation of native type I collagen, by cells resident in the bone. This might be of particular importance in the degradation of the organic bone matrix during the early stages of osteolysis, which has been shown to be both necessary and sufficient to activate osteoclastic bone resorption.

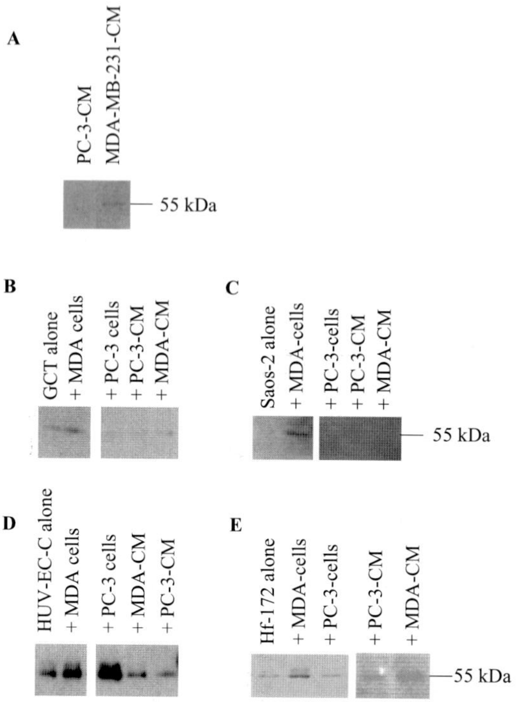

Figure 1. The effect of human bone-metastatic tumor cells on the interstitial collagenase MMP-1 expression in human cells representing stromal components of the bone (monocyte osteoclast-like GCT cells, osteosarcoma osteoblast-like Saos-2 cells, endothelial umbilical vein HUV-EC-C cells, and fibroblast Hf-172 cells). Subconfluent human prostate adenocarcinoma PC-3 and human breast adenocarcinoma MDA-MB-231 cells were incubated in serum-free media for 24 h. The conditioned media were collected and added to subconfluent GCT, Saos-2, HUV-EC-C, or Hf-172 cells for 24 h to constitute up to 50% of the media. Subconfluent GCT, Saos-2, HUV-EC-C, or Hf-172 cells were also co-cultured with MDA-MB-231 and PC-3 cells and their conditioned media were collected over a 24 h-period. Cell number-standardized samples were subjected to 10% SDS-PAGE and subsequent Western blotting to determine protein expression. We used a monoclonal MMP-1 antibody (0.5 □g/ml, Oncogene Research Products, Cambridge, MA) and subsequently a goat anti-mouse antibody conjugated with horseradish peroxidase (HRP) (1:2000, Santa Cruz Biotechnology, Santa Cruz, CA). ECL chemiluminescence detection (Amersham, Canada) was used to visualize the proteins. (A) Western blot analysis for MMP-1 protein. MMP-1 (at 55 kDa) is expressed in 24 h-conditioned media from human bone metastatic breast adenocarcinoma MDA-MB-231 cells, but not from prostate adenocarcinoma PC-3 cells. Lanes 1 in (B), (C), (D), and (E) demonstrate MMP-1 expression in 24 h-conditioned media of the cells representing stromal components of the bone: (B) osteoclast-like GCT cells, (C) osteoblast-like Saos-2 cells, (D) endothelial HUV-EC-C cells, and (E) fibroblast Hf-172 cells. Lanes 2 and 3 show the results of the co-culture (24 h) experiments of PC-3 or MDA-MB-231 cells together with cells representing stromal components of the bone. Protein expression in cells representing stromal components of the bone 24 h after the addition of conditioned media derived from cancer cells (50%) is presented in lanes 4 and 5.

These results support the role of a membrane-bound, inducing factor on the tumor cells, such as EMMPRIN, since the most dramatic increases are observed when cells are co-cultured. However, the expression of EMMPRIN is probably not the only factor affecting the expression of MMPs, since both MDA-MB-231 and PC-3 cells express EMMPRIN (data not shown), but their pattern of induction of MMP expression is different. The observed differences could also be related to the differences in bone metastasis from breast and prostate cancer.

4. MATRIX METALLOPROTEINASE INHIBITORS

During the last decade synthetic MMP inhibitors have been developed for the treatment of cancer. They are able to effectively reduce or prevent the formation of metastases in a number of animal studies. Many MMP inhibitors, including batimastat, marimastat, AG3340 (Prinomastat), and BMS-275291 have been tested in clinical trials for various types of cancer. Unfortunately, most trials were unsuccessful and some were ended prematurely.

Batimastat (BB-94) was the first MMP inhibitor to be tested in cancer patients. It is a peptide-like analogue of the collagen substrate and a broad spectrum MMP inhibitor. *In vitro* studies show that batimastat is able to inhibit basement membrane degradation by human breast cancer cells (172), invasion of various cells into a reconstituted basement membrane (173) and degradation of type IV collagen (174). Batimastat has been shown to reduce the tumor burden of orthotopic xenografts of ovarian, colon, and breast cancer and to inhibit the formation of distant metastases in these murine models (149, 175-177). In a rat mammary carcinoma model batimastat was administered two days prior to surgical removal of primary tumors and continued for 73 days. At 120 days, 100% of the animals were disease-free compared to death in all controls. These results point to a potential for MMP inhibitors as a neoadjuvant or protective mode immediately prior to breast cancer surgery (178). Moreover, batimastat potentiates the activity of cisplatin, the most effective chemotherapy regimen for ovarian cancer patients, in an ovarian carcinoma mouse model (179). Phase I studies in patients with malignant ascites (180) and malignant pleural effusions (181) have been completed for this drug. Batimastat is well tolerated at doses that result in sustained plasma concentrations that are higher than the IC_{50}. Even though the phase I trials showed promising results, batimastat has been discontinued due to poor bioavailability.

Marimastat is a second-generation MMP inhibitor with better oral bioavailability. A meta-analysis using data from dose-finding studies for advanced and serologically progressive cancers on a total of 415 patients shows that there is a significant effect of marimastat on the levels of cancer specific antigens (182). A pilot study of marimastat in advanced gastric cancer patients revealed that marimastat increases the fibrous tissue covering the tumors and decreases the haemorrhagic appearance at day 28 after start of the treatment (183). Phase I studies have also shown that marimastat in combination with chemotherapy agents such as doxorubicin, cyclophosphamide (184), 5-fluoruracil (185) or carboplatin (186) is well tolerated and the combination does not cause additional toxicity. A randomized, double-blind, placebo-controlled study using marimastat in non-resectable gastric cancer demonstrates an increase in both overall and progression-free survival (187).

Other MMP inhibitors, such as BAY 12-9566 and AG3340, reached the stage of phase III clinical trials (188), but were eventually halted. In animals, BAY 12-9566 has shown efficacy in murine models of B16/F10 melanoma and Lewis lung carcinoma (189) and in orthotopic tumor models of human breast cancer (190) and colon carcinoma (191). In combination with doxorubicin, plasma levels of BAY 12-9566 remain the same, however the haematological toxicity seems slightly more pronounced, but is not dose-limiting (192). In 2000, all clinical trials in cancer involving BAY 12-9566 were halted following a recommendation from an independent Data Safety Monitoring Board to close the non-small cell lung cancer trial due to excessive deaths in the BAY 12-9566 arm. AG3340 has been extensively tested in animal studies including the murine B16/F10 melanoma and Lewis lung carcinoma models (193), human malignant glioma (194), and colon adenocarcinoma models (195) and shows a high efficacy in these models, ranging from reduction in primary tumor size, invasion and number of metastases. A combination of AG3340 with carboplatin markedly increases survival of rats bearing human lung cancer xenografts (196). In addition to MMP inhibitory activity, AG3340 also has the potential to inhibit proliferation of human colon adenocarcinoma cells *in vivo* (194, 195) and induce apoptosis in human prostate adenocarcinoma PC-3 cells grown subcutaneously in nude mice (197). After prolonged treatment of animals with AG3340 the tumor-suppressing effect observed initially disappears, however, this does not seem to be due to induced resistance (198-200). Lack of effectiveness of AG3340 was eventually the reason to stop phase III clinical trials in advanced non-small cell lung cancer and prostate cancer.

One MMP inhibitor, BMS-275291, is still under investigation in a phase II trial involving hormone-refractory prostate cancer patients. BMS-275291 is an orally available broad-spectrum MMP inhibitor effective against MMP-1, MMP-2, MMP-7, MMP-9 and MT1-MMP in nanomolar concentrations.

BMS-275291 is able to dose-dependently inhibit lung metastases in mice after intravenous injection of B16/BL6 cells (201).

Furthermore, tetracyclines are potent inhibitors of cancer cell proliferation (202, 209-211), suggesting a direct indication for anti-tumor therapy. We have demonstrated that doxycycline is capable of inhibiting tumor cell growth in a concentration-dependent manner in bone metastasizing cancer cells (Figure 2B). Doxycycline is also able to inhibit MMP-2 and MMP-9 activity by 80% (Figure 2A) (162).

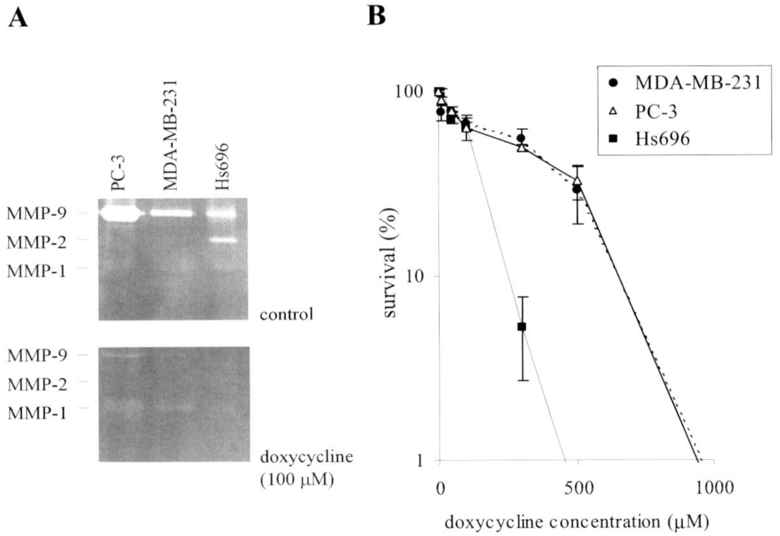

Figure 2. (A) Doxycycline-induced inhibition of MMP activity secreted by bone metastasizing cancer cells. Subconfluent human prostate adenocarcinoma PC-3, human breast adenocarcinoma MDA-MB-231, and Hs696 cells (human adenocarcinoma of unknown primary origin) were incubated in serum-free media for 24 h. The conditioned media were collected, concentrated and samples were subjected to gelatin enzymography to assess MMP-activity. The zymograms were incubated in substrate buffer in the absence (control) or presence of 100 μM doxycycline. Matrix metalloproteinase activity of 92-kDa type IV collagenase (MMP-9) and 72-kDa type IV collagenase (MMP-2) secreted by bone-metastasizing cancer cells was largely abolished by incubation in 100 μM doxycycline. (B) Survival curves of bone metastasizing human cancer cells (PC-3, MDA-MB-231, and Hs696) as measured by colony forming assay in a 24 h-treatment protocol. Values are represented as ratios of treated over corresponding control. Each value represents mean data (± S.E.) of three experiments carried out in triplicate. Mean survival for human prostate adenocarcinoma PC-3 cells treated with 500 μM doxycycline was 0.6±1.0%, for human breast adenocarcinoma MDA-MB-231 and human adenocarcinoma Hs696 cells treated with 1000 μM doxycycline the mean survival amounted to 0.7±0.5 and 0.6±0.0%, respectively. Mean values reached significance ($p<0.05$) for PC-3 cells at 50 μM doxycycline, for MDA-MB-231 and Hs696 cells at 100 μM doxycycline.

5. THE FUTURE OF BONE METASTASIS TREATMENT

A targetted therapy consisting of a combination of bisphophonates, MMP inhibitors, and/or tetracyclines could potentially be more successful. MMP inhibitors that might prove to be useful in cancers with an overexpression of MMP-2 or MMP-9 might actually not be the best approach for therapy of bone metastasis. When the tumors spread to the bone the inhibition of MMPs, such as the interstitial collagenases MMP-1, MMP-8, and MMP-13, might be more beneficial in the reduction or prevention of bone destruction. MMP inhibitors are currently being designed for use in rheumatoid arthritis to prevent bone and cartilage loss. They are more effective against the interstitial collagenases, the same MMPs that are also involved in the breakdown of cartilage components. A combinatory and/or sequential treatment with MMP inhibitors directed towards the interstitial collagenases, such as bisphosphonates, and/or tetracyclines might be beneficial. Further investigation into the potential of combination treatment might be a valuable approach towards the ultimate goal of controlling bone metastasis.

ACKNOWLEDGEMENTS

We would like to thank E. Seidlitz, S. Popovic, Š. Lhoták, and H. Hirte for their assistance. This research was supported by the Canadian Institutes of Health Research and National Cancer Institute of Canada.

LIST OF ABBREVIATIONS:

MMP:	Matrix Metalloproteinase
TIMP:	Tissue Inhibitor of Matrix Mettalloproteinase
EMMPRIN:	Extracellular Matrix Metalloproteinase Inducer

REFERENCES

1. Abrams HL, Spiro R, Goldstein N. Metastases in carcinoma: Analysis of 1000 autopsied cases. Cancer, 3: 74-85, 1950.
2. Tofe AJ, Francis MD, Harvey WJ. Correlation of neoplasms with incidence and localization of skeletal metastases: An analysis of 1355 diphosphate bone scans. J Nucl Med, 16: 986-989, 1975.
3. Kanis JA. Bone and cancer: Pathophysiology and treatment of metastases. Bone, 17: 101S-105S, 1995.
4. Hortobagyi GN. Bone metastases in breast cancer patients. Semin Onco, 18: 11-15, 1991.
5. Moro L, Gazzarrini C, Crivellari D, Galligioni E, Talamini R, de Bernard B. Biochemical markers for detecting bone metastases in patients with breast cancer. Clin Chem, 39: 131-134, 1993.
6. Mundy GR, Roodman GD, Bonewald LF, Orefo RO, Boyce BF. Assays for bone resorption and bone formation. Methods Enzymol, 198: 502-510, 1991.
7. Charhon SA, Chapuy MC, Delvin EE, Valentin-Opran A, Edouard CM., Meunier PJ. Histomorphometric analysis of sclerotic bone metastases from prostatic carcinoma with special reference to osteomalacia. Cancer, 51: 918-924, 1983.
8. Urwin GH, Percival RC, Beneton MNC, Williams JL, Kanis JA. Generalised increase in bone resorption in carcinoma of the prostate. Br J Urol, 57: 721-723, 1985.
9. Maeda H, Koizumi M, Yoshimura K, Yamauchi T, Kawai T, Ogata E. Correlation between bone metabolic markers and bone scan in prostatic cancer. J Urol, 157: 539-543, 1997.
10. Anderson, KC, Lust JA. Role of cytokines in multiple myeloma. Semin Hematol, 36: 14-20, 1999.
11. Vihinen P, Kahari VM. Matrix metalloproteinases in cancer: Prognostic markers and therapeutic targets. Int J Cancer, 99: 157-166, 2002.
12. Egeblad M, Werb Z. New functions for the matrix metalloproteinases in cancer progression. Nat Rev Cancer, 2: 161-174, 2002.
13. Shingleton WD, Hodges DJ, Brick P, Cawston TE. Collagenase: A key enzyme in collagen turnover. Biochem. Cell Biol, 74: 759-775, 1996.
14. Powell WC, Matrisian LM. Complex roles of matrix metalloproteinases in tumor progression. Curr Top Microbiol Immunol, 213: 1-21, 1996.
15. Seiki M. Membrane type-matrix metalloproteinase and tumor invasion. Curr Top Microbiol Immunol, 213: 23-32, 1996.
16. Sato M, Grassner W, Endo N, Atkins R, Simmons H, Thompson DD, Golub E, Rodan G. A. Bisphosphonate action: Alendronate localization in rat bone and effects on osteoclast ultrastructure. J Clin Invest, 88: 2095-2105, 1991.
17. Sato H, Seiki M. Membrane-type matrix metalloproteinases (MT-MMPs) in tumor metastasis. J Biochem, 119: 209-215, 1996.
18. Will H, Hinzmann B. cDNA sequence and mRNA tissue distribution of a novel human matrix metalloproteinase with a potential transmembrane segment. Eur J Biochem, 231: 602-608, 1995.

49. Yu Q, Stamenkovic I. Cell surface-localized matrix metalloproteinase-9 proteolytically activates TGF-beta and promotes tumor invasion and angiogenesis. Genes Dev, 14: 163-176, 2000.
50. Gearing AJH, Beckett P, Christodoulou M, Churchill M, Clements J, Davidson AH, Drummond AH, Galloway WA, Gilbert R, Gordon JL, Leber TM, Mangan M, Miller K, Nayee P, Owen K, Patel S, Thomas W, Wells G, Wood LM, Wooloey K. Processing of tumor necrosis factor-α precursor by metalloproteinases. Nature, 370: 555-557, 1994.
51. Schonbeck U, Mach F, Libby P. Generation of biologically active IL-1 beta by matrix metalloproteinases: a novel caspase-1-independent pathway of IL-1 beta processing. J Immunol, 161: 3340-3346, 1998.
52. Kajita M, Itoh Y, Chiba T, Mori H, Okada A, Kinoh H, Seiki M. Membrane-type 1 matrix metalloproteinase cleaves CD44 and promotes cell migration. J Cell Bio, 153: 893-904, 2001.
53. Okamoto I, Kawano Y, Tsuiki H, Sasaki J, Nakao M, Matsumoto M, Suga M, Ando M, Nakajima M, Saya H. CD44 cleavage induced by a membrane-associated metalloprotease plays a critical role in tumor cell migration. Oncogene, 18: 1435-1446, 1999.
54. Noë V, Fingleton B, Jacobs K, Crawford HC, Vermeulen S, Steelant W, Bruyneel E, Matrisian LM, Mareel M. Release of an invasion promoter E-cadherin fragment by matrilysin and stromelysin-1. J Cell Sci, 114: 111-118, 2001.
55. Giannelli G, Falk-Marzillier J, Schiraldi O, Stetler-Stevenson WG, Quaranta V. Induction of cell migration by matrix metalloproteinase-2 cleavage of laminin-5. Science, 277: 225-228, 1997.
56. Codony-Servat J, Albanell J, Lopez-Talavera JC, Arribas J, Basega J. Cleavage of the HER2 ectodomain is a pervanadate-activable process that is inhibited by the tissue inhibitor of metalloproteinases-1 in breast cancer cells. Cancer Res, 59: 1196-1201, 1999.
57. Hargreaves PG, Wang F, Antcliff J, Murphy G, Lawry J, Russell RGG, Croucher PI. Human myeloma cells shed the interleukin-6 receptor: Inhibition by tissue inhibitor of metalloproteinase-3 and a hydroxamate-based metalloproteinase inhibitor. Br J Haematol, 101: 694-702, 1998.
58. Smith MR, Kung H, Durum SK, Colburn NH, Sun Y. TIMP-3 induces cell death by stabilizing TNF-α receptors on the surface of human colon carcinoma cells. Cytokine, 9: 770-780, 1997.
59. Rivas MJG, Arii S, Furutani M, Harada T, Mizumoto M, Nishiyama H, Fujita J, Imamura M. Expression of human macrophage metalloelastase gene in hepatocellular carcinoma: Correlation with angiostatin generation and its clinical significance. Hepatology, 28: 986-993, 1998.
60. Furcht LT, Skubitz APN, Fields GB. Tumor cell invasion, matrix metalloproteinases, and the dogma. Lab Invest, 70: 781-783, 1994.
61. Liotta LA, Tryggvason K, Garbisa S, Hart IR, Foltz CM, Shafie S. Metastatic potential correlates with enzymatic degradation of basement membrane collagen. Nature, 284: 67-68, 1980.

62. Nakajima M, Welch DR, Belloni PN, Nicolson GL. Degradation of basement membrane type IV collagen and lung subendothelial matrix by rat mammary adenocarcinoma cell clones of differing metastatic potentials. Cancer Res, 47: 4869-4876, 1987.
63. Turpeenniemi-Hujanen T, Thorgeirsson UP, Hart IR, Grant SS, Liotta LA. Expression of collagenase IV (basement membrane collagenase) Activity in murine tumor cell hybrids that differ in metastatic potential. J Natl Cancer Inst, 75: 99-103, 1985.
64. Sreenath T, Matrisian LM, Stetler-Stevenson W, Gattoni-Celli S, Pozzatti RO. Expression of matrix metalloproteinase genes in transformed rat cell lines of high and low metastatic potential. Cancer Res, 52: 4942-4947, 1992.
65. Wilson CL, Heppner KJ, Labosky PA, Hogan BL, Matrisian LM. Intestinal tumorigenesis is suppressed in mice lacking the metalloproteinase matrilysin. Proc Natl Acad Sci USA, 94: 1402-1407, 1997.
66. Masson R, Lefebvre O, Noe A, Fahime ME, Chenard MP, Wendling C, Kebers F, LeMeur M, Dierich A, Foidart JM, Basset P, Rio MC. In vivo evidence that the stromelysin-3 metalloproteinase contributes in a paracrine manner to epithelial cell malignancy. J Cell Biol, 140: 1535-1541, 1998.
67. Udagawa N, Takahashi N, Jimi E, Matsuzaki K, Tsurukai T, Itoh K, Nakagawa N, Yasuda H, Goto M, Tsuda E, Higashio K, Gillespie MT, Martin TJ, Suda T. Osteoblasts/stromal cells stimulate osteoclast activation through expression of osteoclast differentiation factor/RANKL but not macrophage colony-stimulating factor. Bone, 25: 517-523, 1999.
68. Davies B, Miles DW, Happerfield LC, Naylor MS, Bobrow LG, Rubens RD, Balkwill FR. Activity of type IV collagenases in benign and malignant breast disease. Br. J. Cancer, 67: 1126-1131, 1993.
69. Gress TM, Müller-Pillasch F, Lerch MM, Friess H, Büchler M, Adler G. Expression and in-situ localization of genes coding for extracellular matrix proteins and extracellular matrix degrading proteases in pancreatic cancer. Int J Cancer, 62: 407-413, 1995.
70. Boag AH, Young ID. Immunohistochemical analysis of type IV collagenase expression in prostatic hyperplasia and adenocarcinoma. Mod Pathol, 6: 65-68, 1993.
71. Hamdy FC, Fadlon EJ, Cottam D, Lawry J, Thurrell W, Silcocks PB, Anderson JB, Williams JL, Rees RC. Matrix metalloproteinase 9 expression in primary human prostatic adenocarcinoma and benign prostatic hyperplasia. Br J Cancer, 69: 177-182, 1994.
72. Tamakoshi K, Kikkawa F, Nawa A, Ishikawa H, Mizuno K, Tamakoshi A, Yamagata S, Suganuma N, Tomoda Y. Characterization of extracellular matrix-degrading proteinase and its inhibitor in gynecologic cancer tissues with clinically different metastatic form. Cancer, 76: 2565-2571, 1995.
73. Takemura M, Azuma C, Kimura T, Kanai T, Saji F, Tanizawa O. Type-IV collagenase and tissue inhibitor of metalloproteinase in ovarian cancer tissues. Int J Gynaecol Obstet, 46: 303-309, 1994.
74. Davies B, Waxman J, Wasan H, Abel P, Williams G, Krausz T, Neal D, Thomas D, Hanby A, Balkwill F. Levels of matrix metalloproteinase in bladder cancer correlate with tumor grade and invasion. Cancer Res, 53: 5365-5369, 1993.

75. Davidson B, Goldberg I, Kopolovic J, Lerner-Geva L, Gotlieb WH, Weis B, Ben-Baruch G, Reich R. Expression of matrix metalloproteinase-9 in squamous cell carcinoma of the uterine cervix-Clinicopathologic study using immunohistochemistry and mRNA in situ hybridization. Gynecol Oncol, 72: 380-386, 1999.
76. Arii S, Mise M, Harada T, Furutani M, Ishigami SI, Niwano M, Mizumoto M, Fukumoto M, Imamura M. Overexpression of matrix metalloproteinase 9 gene in hepatocellular carcinoma with invasive potential. Hepatology, 24: 316-322, 1996.
77. Hewitt RE, Leach IH, Powe DG, Clark IM, Cawston TE, Turner DR. Distribution of collagenase and tissue inhibitor of metalloproteinases (TIMP) in colorectal tumors. Int J Cancer, 49: 666-672, 1991.
78. van der Stappen JW, Hendriks T, Wobbes T. Correlation between collagenolytic activity and grade of histological differentiation in colorectal tumors. Int J Cancer, 45: 1071-1078, 1990.
79. Murray GI, Duncan ME, O'Neil P, Melvin WT, Fothergill JE. Matrix metalloproteinase-1 is associated with poor prognosis in colorectal cancer. Nature Med, 2: 461-462, 1996.
80. Muller D, Breathnach R, Engelmann A, Millon R, Bronner G, Flesch H, Dumont P, Eber M, Abecassis J. Expression of collagenase-related metalloproteinase genes in human lung or head and neck tumors. Int J Cancer, 48: 550-556, 1991.
81. Nakapoulou L, Giannopoulou I, Gakiopoulou H, Liapis H, Tzonou A, Davaris PS. Matrix metalloproteinase-1 and -3 in breast cancer: Correlation with progesterone receptors and other clinicopathologic features. Hum Pathol, 30: 436-442, 1999.
82. Freije JM, Diez-Itza I, Balbin M, Sanchez LM, Blasco R, Tolivia J, López-Otín C. Molecular cloning and expression of collagenase-3, a novel human metalloproteinase produced by breast carcinomas. J Biol Chem, 269: 16766-16773, 1994.
83. Ring P, Johansson K, Höyhtyä M, Rubin K, Lindmark G. Expression of tissue inhibitor of metalloproteinases TIMP-2 in human colorectal cancer-A predictor of tumor stage. Br J Cancer, 76: 805-811, 1997.
84. Johansson N, Vaalamo M, Grénman S, Hietanen S, Klemi P, Saarialho-Kere U, Kähäri VM. Collagenase-3 (MMP-13) is expressed by tumor cells in invasive squamous cell carcinomas. Am J Pathol, 154: 469-480, 1999.
85. Linder C, Engel G, Auer G, Strander H, Linder S. Distribution of stromelysin-3 mRNA transcripts and microvessels in human breast carcinoma. Breast Cancer Res Treat, 42: 207-213, 1997.
86. Chenard MP, O'Siorain L, Shering S, Rouyer N, Lutz Y, Wolf C, Basset P, Bellocq JP, Duffy MJ. High levels of stromelysin-3 correlate with poor prognosis in patients with breast carcinoma. Int J Cancer, 69: 448-451, 1996.
87. Pajouh MS, Nagle RB, Breathnach R, Finch JS, Brawer MK, Bowden GT. Expression of metalloproteinase genes in human prostate cancer. J Cancer Res Clin Onco., 117: 144-150, 1991.
88. Campo E, Merino MJ, Tavassoli FA, Charonis AS, Stetler-Stevenson WG., Liotta LA. Evaluation of basement membrane components and the 72 kDa type IV collagenase in serous tumors of the ovary. Am J Surg Pathol, 16: 500-507, 1992.

89. Autio-Harmainen H, Karttunen T, Hurskainen T, Höyhtyä M, Kauppila A, Tryggvason K. Expression of 72 kilodalton type IV collagenase (gelatinase A) in benign and malignant ovarian tumors. Lab Inves, 69: 312-321, 1993.
90. Stearns M, Wang M. Type IV collagenase (Mr 72,000) expression in human prostate: benign and malignant tissue. Cancer Res, 53: 878-883, 1993.
91. Levy AT, Cioce V, Sobel ME, Garbisa S, Grignioni WF, Liotta LA, Stetler-Stevenson WG. Increased expression of the Mr 72,000 type IV collagenase in human colonic adenocarcinoma. Cancer Res, 51: 439-444, 1991.
92. Ueno H, Nakamura H, Inoue M, Imai K, Noguchi M, Sato H, Seiki M, Okada Y. Expression and tissue localization of membrane-types 1, 2 and 3 matrix metalloproteinases in human invasive breast cancer carcinomas. Cancer Res, 57: 2055-2060, 1997.
93. Nakamura H, Ueno H, Yamashita K, Shimada T, Yamamoto E, Noguchi M, Fujimoto N, Sato H, Seik M, Okada Y. Enhanced production and activation of progelatinase A mediated by membrane type 1 matrix metalloproteinase in human papillary thyroid carcinomas. Cancer Res, 59: 467-473, 1999.
94. Caenazzo C, Onisto M, Sartor L, Scalerta R, Giraldo A, Nitti D, Garbisa S. Augmented membrane type 1 matrix metalloproteinase (MT1-MMP):MMP-2 messenger RNA ratio in gastric carcinomas with poor prognosis. Clin Cancer Res, 4: 2179-2186, 1998.
95. Nomura H, Sato H, Seiki M, Mai M, Okada Y. Expression of membrane-type matrix metalloproteinase in human gastric carcinomas. Cancer Res, 55: 3263-3266, 1995.
96. Mori M, Mimori K, Shiraishi T, Fujie T, Baba K, Kusumoto H, Haraguchi,M, Ueo H, Akiyoshi T. Analysis of MT1-MMP and MMP-2 expression in human gastric cancers. Int J Cancer, 74: 316-321, 1997.
97. Yamamoto M, Mohanam S, Sawaya R, Fuller GN, Seiki M, Sato H, Gokaslan ZL, Liotta LA, Nicolson GL, Rao JS. Differential expression of membrane-type matrix metalloproteinase and its correlation with gelatinase A activation in human malignant brain tumors in vivo and in vitro. Cancer Res, 56: 384-392, 1996.
98. Harada T, Arii S, Mise M, Imamura T, Higashitsuji H, Furutani M, Niwano M, Ishigami SI, Fukumoto M, Seiki M, Sato H, Imamura M. Membrane-type matrix metalloprotainase-1 (MT1-MMP) gene is overexpressed in highly invasive hepatocellular carcinomas. J Hepato, 28: 231-239, 1998.
99. Ogata R, Torimura T, Kin M, Ueno T, Tateishi Y, Kuromatsu R, Shimauchi Y, Sakamoto M, Tamak S, Sata M, Tanikawa K. Increased expression of membrane type 1 matrix metalloproteinase and matrix metalloproteinase-2 with tumor dedifferentiation in hepatocellular carcinomas. Hum Pathol, 30: 443-450, 1999.
100. Nuovo GJ, MacConnell PB, Simsir A, Valea F, French DL. Correlation of the in situ detection of polymerase chain reaction-amplified metalloproteinase complementary DNAs and their inhibitors with prognosis in cervical cancer. Cancer Res, 55: 267-275, 1995.
101. Alvarez OA, Carmichael DF, DeClerck YA. Inhibition of collagenolytic activity and metastasis of tumor cells by a recombinant human tissue inhibitor of metalloproteinases. J Natl Cancer Inst, 82: 589-595, 1990.

102. Khokha R. Suppression of the tumorigenic and metastatic abilities of murine B16-F10 melanoma cels in vivo by the overexpression of the tissue inhibitor of the metalloproteinases-1. J Natl Cancer Inst, 86: 299-304, 1994.
103. DeClerck YA, Perez N, Shimada H, Boone TC, Langley KE, Taylor SM. Inhibition of invasion and metastasis in cells transfected with an inhibitor of metalloproteinases. Cancer Res, 52: 701-708, 1992.
104. Testa JE. Loss of metastatic phenotype by a human epidermoid carcinoma cell line, HEp-3, is accompanied by increased expression of tissue inhibitor of metalloproteinase-2. Cancer Res, 52: 5597-5603, 1992.
105. Moses MA. The regulation of neovascularization by matrix metalloproteinases and their inhibitors. Stem Cells, 15: 180-189, 1997.
106. Ahonen M, Baker AH, Kähär VM. Adenovirus-mediated gene delivery of tissue inhibitor of metalloproteinases-3 inhibits invasion and induces apoptosis in melanoma cells. Cancer Res, 58: 2310-2315, 1998.
107. Wang M, Liu YE, Greene J, Sheng S, Fuchs A, Rosen EM, Shi YE. Inhibition of tumor growth and metastasis of human breast cancer cells transfected with tissue inhibitor of metalloproteinase 4. Oncogene, 14: 2767-2774, 1997.
108. Anand-Apte B, Bao L, Smith R, Iwata K, Olsen BR, Zetter B, Apte SS. A review of tissue inhibitor of metalloproteinase-3 (TIMP-3) and experimental analysis of its effect on primary tumor growth. Biochem Cell Biol, 74: 853-862, 1996.
109. Yoneda T, Sasaki A, Dunstan C, Williams PJ, Bauss F, DeClerck YA, Mundy, GR. Inhibition of osteolytic bone metastasis of breast cancer by combined treatment with the bisphosphonate Ibandronate and tissue inhibitor of the matrix metalloproteinase-2. J Clin Invest, 99: 2509-2517, 1997.
110. Stearns M, Wang M. Immunoassays of the metalloproteinase (MMP-2) and tissue inhibitor of metalloproteinase (TIMPs 1 and 2) levels in noninvasive and metastatic PC-3 clones: Effects of taxol. Oncol Res, 6: 195-201, 1994.
111. Lokeshwar BL, Selze MG, Block NL, Gunja-Smisth Z. Secretion of matrix metalloproteinases and their inhibitors (tissue inhibitor of metalloproteinases) by human prostate in explant cultures: Reduced tissue inhibitor of metalloproteinase secretion by malignant tissues. Cancer Res, 53: 4493-4498, 1993.
112. Grigioni WF, D'Errico A, Fortunato C, Fiorentino M, Mancini AM, Stetler-Stevenson, WG, Sobel ME, Liotta LA, Onisto M, Garbisa S. Prognosis of gastric carcinoma revealed by interactions between tumor cells and basement membrane. Mod Pathol, 7: 220-225, 1994.
113. Ko BK, Cho HR, Choi DW, Nam CW, Park CJ, Kim GY, Kim SS, Woo YJ, Huh J, Lim MY. Reduced expression of tissue inhibitor of metalloproteinase in nodal metastasis of stomach cancer. J Korean Med Sci, 13: 286-290, 1998.
114. Wagner SN, Ockenfels HM, Wagner C, Soyer HP, Goos M. Differential expression of tissue inhibitor of metalloproteinases-2 by cutaneous sqaumous and basal cell carcinomas. J Invest Dermatol, 106: 321-326, 1996.
115. Kikkawa F, Tamakoshi K, Nawa A, Shibata K, Yamagata S, Yamagata T, Suganuma N. Positive correlation between inhibitors of matrix metalloproteinase 1 and matrix metalloproteinases in malignant ovarian tumor tissues. Cancer Lett, 120: 109-115, 1997.

116. Sh Y, Parhar RS, Zou M, Hammami MM, Akhtar M, Lum ZP, Farid NR, Al Sedairy ST, Paterson MC. Tissue inhibitor of metalloproteinases-1 (TIMP-1) mRNA is elevated in advanced stages of thyroid carcinoma. Br J Cancer, 79: 1234-1239, 1999.
117. Ree AH, Flørenes VA, Berg JP, Mælandsmo GM, Nesland JM, Fodstad Ø. High levels of messenger RNAs for tissue inhibitors of metalloproteinases (TIMP-1 and TIMP-2) in primary breast carcinomas are associated with development of distant metastases. Clin Cancer Res, 3: 1623-1628, 1997.
118. Zeng ZS, Cohen AM, Zhang ZF, Stetler-Stevenson W, Guillem JG. Elevated tissue inhibitor of metalloproteinase 1 RNA in colorectal cancer stroma correlates with lymph node and distant metastases. Clin Cancer Res, 1: 899-906, 1995.
119. Lu X, Levy M, Weisnstein B, Santella RM. Immunological quantitation of levels of tissue inhibitor of metalloproteinase-1 in human colon cancer. Cancer Res, 51: 6231-6235, 1991.
120. Kallakury BV, Karikehalli S, Haholu A, Sheehan CE, Azumi N, Ros, JS. Increased expression of matrix metalloproteinases 2 and 9 and tissue inhibitors of metalloproteinases 1 and 2 correlate with poor prognostic variables in renal cell carcinoma. Clin Cancer Res, 7: 3113-3119, 2001.
121. Hayakawa T, Yamashita K, Tanzawa K, Uchijima E, Iwata K. Growth-promoting activity of tissue inhibitor of metalloproteinases-1 (TIMP-1) for a wide range of cells. FEBS Lett, 298: 29-32, 1992.
122. Nemeth JA, Goolsby CL. TIMP-2, a growth-stimulatory protein from SV-40-transformed human fibroblasts. Exp Cell Res, 207: 376-382, 1993.
123. Guedez L, Stetler-Stevenson WG, Wolff L, Wang J, Fukushima P, Mansoor A, Stetler-Stevenson M. In vitro suppression of programmed cell death of B cells by tissue inhibitor of metalloproteinases-1. J Clin Invest, 102: 2002-2010, 1998.
124. Li G, Fridman R, Kim HR. Tissue inhibitor of metalloproteinase-1 inhibits apoptosis of human breast epithelial cells. Cancer Res, 59: 6267-6275, 1999.
125. Valente P, Fassina G, Melchiori A, Masiello L, Cilli M, Vacca A, Onisto M, Santi L, Stetler-Stevenson WG, Albini A. TIMP-2 over-expression reduces invasion and angiogenesis and protects B16F10 melanoma cells from apoptosis. Int J Cancer, 75: 246-253, 1998.
126. Jiang Y, Goldberg ID, Shi YE. Complex roles of tissue inhibitors of metalloproteinases in cancer. Oncogene, 21: 2245-2252, 2002.
127. Green J. The physicochemical structure of bone: Cellular and noncellular elements. Miner. Electrolyte Metab, 20: 7-15, 1994.
128. Koop S, MacDonald IC, Luzzi K, Schmidt EE, Morris VL, Grattan M, Khokha R, Chambers AF, Groom AC. Fate of melanoma cells entering the microcirculation: Over 80% survive and extravasate. Cancer Res, 55: 2520-2523, 1995.
129. Chambers TJ, Fuller K. Bone cells predispose bone surfaces to resorption by exposure of mineral to osteoclastic contact. J Cell Sci, 76: 155-165, 1985.
130. Athanasou NA, Wells CA, Quinn J, Heryet A, McGee JO. The origin and nature of stromal osteoclast-like multinucleated giant cells in breast carcinoma: Implications for tumor osteolysis and macrophage biology. Br J Cancer, 59: 491-498, 1989.

131. Taube T, Elomaa I, Blomqvist C, Beneton MNC, Kanis JA. Histomorphometric evidence for osteoclast-mediated bone resorption in metastatic breast cancer. Bone, 15: 161-166, 1994.
132. Galasko CSB. Mechansims of bone destruction in the development of skeletal metastases. Nature, 263: 507-508, 1976.
133. Quinn JMW, McGee JO, Athanasou NA. Human tumor-associated macrophages differentiate into osteoclastic bone-resorbing cells. J Pathol, 184: 31-36, 1998.
134. Sanchez-Sweatman OH, Orr FW, Singh G. Human metastatic prostate PC3 cell lines degrade bone using matrix metalloproteinases. Invasion Metastasis, 18: 297-305, 1999.
135. Bossard MJ, Tomaszek TA, Thompson SK, Amegadzie BY, Hanning CR, Jones C, Kurdyla JT, McNulty DE, Drake FH, Gowen M, Levy MA. Proteolytic activity of human osteoclast cathepsin K. J Biol Chem, 271: 12517-12524, 1996.
136. Drake FH, Dodds RA, James IE, Connor JR, Debouck C, Richardson S, Lee-Rykaczewski E, Coleman L, Rieman D, Barthlow R, Hastings G, Gowen M. Cathepsin K, but not cathepsins B, L, or S, is abundantly expressed in human osteoclasts. J Biol Chem, 271: 12511-12516, 1996.
137. Stahle-Bäckdahl M, Sandstedt B, Bruce K, Lindahl A, Jimenez MG, Vega JA, López-Otín C. Collagenase-3 (MMP-13) is expressed during human fetal ossification and re-expressed in postnatal bone remodeling and rheumatoid arthritis. Lab Invest, 76: 717-728, 1997.
138. Aimes RT, Quigley JP. Matrix metalloproteinase-2 is an interstitial collagenase. J Biol Chem, 270: 5872-5876, 1995.
139. Woessner JF Jr. The family of matrix metalloproteinases. Ann NY Acad Sci, 732: 11-21, 1994.
140. Meikle MC, Bord S, Hembry RM, Reynolds JJ. The synthesis of collagenase, gelatinase-A (72 kDa) and -B (95 kDa), and TIMP-1 and -2 by human osteoblasts from normal and arthritic bone. Bone, 17: 255-260, 1995.
141. Bord S, Horner A, Hembry RM, Reynolds JJ, Compston JE. Production of collagenase by human osteoblasts and osteoclasts in vivo. Bone, 19: 35-40, 1996.
142. Okada Y, Naka K, Kawamura K, Matsumoto T, Nakanishi I, Fujimoto N, Sato H, Seiki M. Localization of matrix metalloproteinase 9 (92-kilodalton gelatinase/type IV collagenase gelatinase B) in osteoclasts: Implications for bone resorption. Lab Invest, 72: 311-322, 1995.
143. Lhotak S, Elavathi LJ, Vukmirovic-Popovic S, Duivenvoorden WC, Tozer RG, Singh G. Immunolocalization of matrix metalloproteinases and their inhibitors in clinical specimens of bone metastasis from breast carcinoma. Clin Exp Metastasis, 18: 463-470, 2000.
144. Basset P, Bellocq JP, Wolf C, Stoll I, Hutin P, Limacher JM, Podhajcer OL, Chenard MP, Rio MC, Chambon P. A novel metalloproteinase gene specifically expressed in stromal cells of breast carcinomas. Nature, 348: 699-704, 1990.
145. Okada A, Bellocq JP, Rouyer N, Chenard MP, Rio MC, Chambon P, Basset P. Membrane-type matrix metalloproteinase (MT-MMP) gene is expressed in stromal cells of human colon, breast, and head and neck carcinomas. Proc Natl Acad Sci USA, 92: 2730-2734, 1995.

146. Polette M, Nawrocki B, Gilles C, Sato H, Seiki M, Tournier JM, Birembaut P. MT-MMP expression and localization in human lung and breast cancers. Virchows Arch, 428: 29-35, 1996.
147. Poulsom R, Hanby AM, Pignatelli M, Jeffery RE, Longcroft JM, Rogers L, Stamp GWH. Expression of gelatinase A and TIMP-2 mRNAs in desmoplastic fibroblasts in both mammary carcinomas and basal cell carcinomas of the skin. J Clin Pathol, 46: 429-436, 1993.
148. Soini Y, Hurskainen T, Höyhtyä M, Oikarinen A, Autio-Harmainen H. 72 KD and 92 KD type IV collagenase, type IV collagen, and laminin mRNAs in breast cancer: A study by in situ hybridization. J Histochem Cytochem, 42: 945-951, 1994.
149. Davies B, Brown PD, East N, Crimmin MJ, Balkwill FR. A synthetic matrix metalloproteinase inhibitor decreases tumor burden and prolongs survival of mice bearing human ovarian carcinoma xenografts. Cancer Res, 53: 2087-2091, 1993.
150. Monteagudo C, Merino MJ, San-Juan J, Liotta LA, Stetler-Stevenson WG. Immunohistochemical distribution of type IV collagenase in normal, benign, and malignant breast tissue. Am J Pathol, 136: 585-592, 1990.
151. Visscher DW, Höyhtyä M, Ottosen SK, Liang CM, Sarkar FH, Crissman JD, Fridman R. Enhanced expression of tissue inhibitor of metalloproteinase-2 (TIMP-2) in the stroma of breast carcinomas correlates with tumor recurrence. Int J Cancer, 59: 339-344, 1994.
152. Basset P, Wolf C, Chambon P. Expression of the stromelysin-3 gene in fibroblastic cells of invasive carcinoma of the breast and other human tissues: A review. Breast Cancer Res Treat, 24: 185-193, 1993.
153. Nielsen BS, Sehested M, Kjeldsen L, Borregaard N, Rygaard J, Danø K. Expression of matrix metalloproteinase-9 in vascular pericytes in human breast cancer. Lab Invest, 77: 345-355, 1997.
154. Montironi R, Lucarini G, Castaldini C, Galluzzi CM, Biagini G, Fabris G. Immunohistochemical evaluation of type IV collagenase (72-Kd metalloproteinase) in prostatic intraepithelial neoplasia. Anticancer Res, 16: 2057-2062, 1996.
155. Varani J, Hattori Y, Dame MK, Schmidt T, Murphy HS, Johnson KJ, Wojno KJ. Matrix metalloproteinases (MMPs) in fresh human prostate tumor tissue and organ-cultured prostate tissue: levels of collagenolytic and gelatinolytic MMPs are low, variable and different in fresh tissue versus organ-cultured tissue. Br J Cancer, 84: 1076-1083, 2001.
156. Barillé S, Akhoundi C, Collette M, Mellerin MP, Rapp MJ, Harousseau JL, Bataille R, Amiot M. Metalloproteinases in multiple myeloma: Production of matrix metalloproteinase-9 (MMP-9), activation of proMMP-2, and induction of MMP-1 by myeloma cells. Blood, 4: 1649-1655, 1997.
157. Clohisy DR, Perkins SL, Ramnaraine MLR. Review of cellular mechanisms of tumor osteolysis. Clin Orthop Rel Res, 373: 104-114, 2000.
158. Clohisy DR, Palkert D, Ramnaraine MLR, Pekurovsky I, Oursler MJ. Human breast cancer induces osteoclast activation and increases the number of osteoclasts at sites of tumor osteolysis. J Orthop Res, 14: 396-402, 1996.
159. Perkel VS, Mohan S, Herring SJ, Baylink,DJ, Linkhart TA. Human prostatic cancer cells, PC3, elaborate mitogenic activity which selectively stimulates human bone cells. Cancer Res, 50: 6902-6907, 1990.

160. Lehr JE, Pienta KJ. Preferential adhesion of prostate cancer cells to a human bone marrow endothelial cell line. J Natl Cancer Inst, 90: 118-123, 1998.
161. Festuccia C, Teti A, Bianco P, Guerra F, Vicentini C, Tennina R, Villanova I, Sciortino G, Bologna M. Human prostatic tumor cells in culture produce growth and differentiation factors active on osteoblasts: a new biological and clinical parameter for prostatic carcinoma. Oncol Res, 9: 419-431, 1997.
162. Duivenvoorden WCM, Hirte HW, Singh G. Use of tetracycline as an inhibitor of matrix metalloproteinase activity secreted by human bone-metastasizing cancer cells. Invasion Metastasis, 17: 312-322, 1997.
163. Brown PD, Levy AT, Margulies IMK, Liotta LA, Stetler-Stevenson WG. Independent expression and cellular processing of Mr 72,000 type IV collagenase and interstitial collagenase in human tumorigenic cell lines. Cancer Res, 50: 6184-6191, 1990.
164. Ohishi K, Fujita N, Moringa Y, Tsuruo T. H-31 human breast cancer cells stimulate type I collagenase production in osteoblast-like cells and induce bone resorption. Clin Exp Metastasis, 13: 287-295, 1995.
165. Lacroix M, Siwek B, Marie PJ, Body JJ. Production and regulation of interleukin-11 by breast cancer cells. Cancer Lett, 127: 29-35, 1998.
166. Utoguchi N, Mizuguchi H, Dantakean A, Makimoto H, Wakai Y, Tsututsumi Y, Nakagawa S, Mayumi T. Effect of tumor cell-conditioned medium on endothelial macromolecular permeability and its correlation with collagen. Br J Cancer, 73: 24-28, 1996.
167. Polette M, Gilles C, Marchand V, Lorenzato M, Toole B, Tournier JM, Zucker S, Birembaut P. Tumor collagenase stimulatory factor (TCSF) expression and localization in human lung and breast cancers. J Histochem Cytochem, 45: 703-709, 1997.
168. Ellis SM, Nabeshima K, Biswas C. Monoclonal antibody preparation and purification of a tumor cell collagenase-stimulatory factor. Cancer Res, 49: 3385-3391, 1989.
169. Rodan SB, Imai Y, Thiede MA, Wesolowski G, Thompson D, Bar-Shavit Z, Shuli S, Mann K, Rodan GA. Characterization of a human osteosarcoma cell line (Saos-2) with osteoblastic properties. Cancer Res, 47: 4961-4966, 1987.
170. DiPerso JF, Brennan JK, Lichtman MA, Speiser BL. Human cell lines that elaborate colony-stimulating activity for the marrow cells of man and other species. Blood, 51: 507-519, 1978.
171. Hoshi H, McKeehan WL. Brain- and liver cell-derived factors are required for growth of human endothelial cells in serum-free culture. Proc Natl Acad Sci USA, 81: 6413-6417, 1984.
172. Stonelake PS, Jones CE, Neoptolemos JP, Baker PR. Proteinase inhibitors reduce basement membrane degradation by human breast cancer cell lines. B. J Cancer, 75: 951-959, 1997.
173. Kolkhorst V, Stürzebecher J, Wiederanders B. Inhibition of tumor cell invasion by protease inhibitors: Correlation with protease profile. J Cancer Res Clin Oncol, 124: 598-606, 1998.
174. Ferry G, Boutin JA, Hennig P, Genton A, Desmet C, Fauchère JL, Atassi G, Tucker GC. A zinc chelator inhibiting gelatinases exerts potent in vitro anti-invasive effects. Eur J Pharmacol, 351: 225-233, 1998.

175. Watson SA, Morris TM, Robinson G, Crimmin MJ, Brown PD, Hardcastle JD. Inhibition of organ invasion by the matrix metalloproteinase inhibitor Batimastat (BB-94) in two human colon carcinoma metastasis models. Cancer Res, 55: 3629-3633, 1995.
176. Wang X, Fu X, Brown PD, Crimmin MJ, Hoffman RM. Matrix metalloproteinase inhibitor BB-94 (Batimastat) inhibits human colon tumor growth and spread in a patient-like orthotopic model in nude mice. Cancer Res, 54: 4726-4728, 1994.
177. Sledge GW Jr, Qulali M, Goulet R, Bone EA, Fife R. Effect of matrix metalloproteinase inhibitor batimastat on breast cancer regrowth and metastasis in athymic mice. J Natl Cancer Inst, 87: 1546-1550, 1995.
178. Eccles SA, Box GM, Court WJ, Bone EA, Thomas W, Brown P. Control of lymphatic and hematogenous metastasis of a rat mammary carcinoma by the matrix metalloproteinase inhibitor Batimastat (BB94). Cancer Res, 56: 2815-2822, 1996.
179. Giavazzi R, Garofalo A, Ferri C, Lucchini V, Bone EA, Chiara S, Brown PD, Nicoletti MI, Taraboletti G. Batimastat, a synthetic inhibitor of matrix metalloproteinases, potentiates the antitumor activity of cisplatin in ovarian carcinoma xenografts. Clin Cancer Res, 4: 985-992, 1998.
180. Beattie GJ, Smyth JF. Phase I study of intraperitoneal metalloproteinase inhibitor BB-94 in patients with malignant ascites. Clin Cancer Res, 4: 1899-1902, 1998.
181. Macaulay VM, O'Byrne KJ, Saunders MP, Braybrooke JP, Long L, Gleeson F, Mason CS, Harris AL, Brown P, Talbot DC. Phase I study of intrapleural Batimastat (BB-94), a matrix metalloproteinase inhibitor, in the treatment of malignant pleural effusions. Clin Cancer Res, 5: 513-520, 1999.
182. Nemunaitis J, Poole C, Primrose J, Rosemurgy A, Melfetano J, Brown P, Berrington A, Cornish A, Lynch K, Rasmussen H, Kerr D, Cox D, Millar A. Combined analysis of studies of the effects of the matrix metalloproteinase inhibitor marimastat on serum tumor markers in advanced cancer: Selection of a biologically active and tolerable dose for longer-term studies. Clin Cancer Res, 4: 1101-1109, 1998.
183. Tierney GM, Griffin NR, Stuart RC, Kasem H, Lynch KP, Lury JT, Brown PD, Millar AW, Steele RJC, Parsons SL. A pilot study of the safety and the effects of the matrix metalloproteinase inhibitor marimastat in gastric cancer. Eur J Cancer, 35: 563-568, 1999.
184. Gradishar W, Sparano J, Cobleigh M, Kennedy MJ, Schuchter L, Wicks L, Rasmussen H. A phase I study of marimastat in combination with doxorubicin and cycloposphamide in patients with metastatic breast cancer. (Abst) Proc Am Soc Clin Oncol 17: 144a, 1998.
185. O'Reilly S, Mani S, Ratain MJ, Elza Brown K, Johnson S, Vogelzang NJ, Kennedy MJ, Donehower R, Rugg T. Schedules of 5FU and the matrix metalloproteinase inhibitor marimastat (MAR): A phase I study. (Abst) Proc Am Soc Clin Oncol, 17: 217a, 1998.
186. Adams M, Thomas H. A phase I study of the matrix metalloproteinase inhibitor, Marimastat, administered concurrently with carboplatin, to patients with relapsed ovarian cancer. (Abst) Proc Am Soc Clin Oncol, 17: 217a, 1998.
187. Bramhall SR, Hallissey MT, Whiting J, Scholefield J, Tierney G, Stuart, RC, Hawkins RE, McCulloch P, Maughan T, Brown PD, Baillet M, Fielding JW. Marimastat as

maintenance therapy for patients with advanced gastric cancer: a randomised trial. Br J Cancer, 86: 1864-1870, 2002.
188. Nelson NJ. Inhibitors of angiogenesis enter phase III testing. J Natl Cancer Inst, 90: 960-963, 1998.
189. Bull C, Flynn C, Eberwein D, Casazza AM, Carter CA, Hibner B. Activity of the biphenyl matrix metalloproteinase inhibitor BAY 12-9566 in murine in vivo models. Proc. Am. Assoc. Cancer Res, 39: 302, 1998.
190. Nozaki S, Sissons S, Casazza AM, Sledge GW Jr. Inhibition of human breast cancer regrowth and pulmonary metastases by BAY 12-9566 in athymic mice. (Abst) Proc Am Assoc Cancer Res, 39: 301, 1998.
191. Flynn C, Bull C, Eberwein D, Matherne C, Hibner B. Anti-metastatic activity of BAY 12-9566 in a human colon carcinoma HCT116 orthotopic model. (Abst) Proc Am Assoc Cancer Res, 39: 301, 1998.
192. Chouinard E, Goel R, Hirte HW, Stewart D, Hurak S, Waterfield B, Matthews S, Elias I, Seymour L. A phase I interaction study between BAY 12-9566 and doxorubicin in cancer patients. (Abst) Proc Am Assoc Cancer Res, 40: 84, 1999.
193. Santos O, McDermott CD, Daniels RG, Appelt K. Rodent pharmacokinetic and anti-tumor efficacy studies with a series of synthetic inhibitors of matrix metalloproteinases. Clin Exp Metastasis, 15: 499-508, 1997.
194. Price A, Shi Q, Morris D, Wilcox ME, Brasher PMA, Rewcastle NB, Shalinsky D, Zou H, Appelt K, Johnston RN, Yong VW, Edwards D, Forsyth P. Marked inhibition of tumor growth in a malignant glioma tumor model by a novel synthetic matrix metalloproteinase inhibitor AG3340. Clin Cancer Res, 5: 845-854, 1999.
195. Shalinsky D, Brekken J, Zou H, McDermott CD, Forsyth P, Edwards DR, Margosiak S, Bender S, Truitt G, Wood A, Varki NM, Appelt, K. Broad antitumor and antiangiogenic activities of AG3340, a potent and selective MMP inhibitor undergoing advanced oncology clinical trials. Ann NY Acad Sci, 878: 236-270, 1998.
196. Johnston MR, Mullen JM, Pagura M, Brekken J, Zou H, Shalinsky D. AG3340 and carboplatin increase survival in an orthotopic nude rat model of primary and metastatic human lung cancer. (Abst) Proc Am Assoc Cancer Res, 40: 293, 1999.
197. Shalinsky D, Brekken J, Zou H, Bender S, Zook S, Appelt K, Webber S, Varki NV. Increased apoptosis in human androgen-independent prostatic PC-3 tumors following oral administration of a novel matrix metalloproteinase (MMP) inhibitor, AG3340, in male nude mice. (Abst) Proc Am Assoc Cancer Res, 39: 646, 1998.
198. Zou H, Brekken J, Shalinsky D. Human tumors retain sensitivity to AG3340, a selective metalloproteinase inhibitor, after extended treatment and serial passage in vivo. (Abst) Proc Am Assoc Cancer Res, 40, 709. 1999.
199. Hibner B, Card A, Flynn C, Casazza AM, Taraboletti G, Rieppi M, Giavazzi R. BAY 12-9566, a novel, biphenyl matrix metalloproteinase inhibitor, demonstrates anti-invasive and anti-angiogenic properties. (Abst) Proc Am Assoc Cancer Res, 39: 302, 1998.
200. Shalinsky D, Zou H, McDermott CD, Brekken J, Niesman MR, Rivero ME, Garcia CR, Freeman MR, Appelt K. AG3340, a selective MMP inhibitor, has broad antiangiogenic activity across oncology and ophthalmology models in vivo. (Abst) Proc Am Assoc Cancer Res, 40: 66, 1999.

201. Naglich JG, Jure-Kunkel M, Gupta E, Fargnoli J, Henderson AJ, Lewin AC, Talbott R, Baxter A, Bird J, Savopoulos R, Wills R, Kramer RA, Trail PA. Inhibition of angiogenesis and metastasis in two murine models by the matrix metalloproteinase inhibitor, BMS-275291. Cancer Res, 61: 8480-8485, 2001.
202. Gordon JM, Walker, CB, Murphy JC, Goodson JM, Socransky SS. Tetracycline: Levels achievable in gingival crevice fluid and in vitro effect on subgingival organisms. Part I. Concentrations in crevical fluid after repeated doses. J Periodont, 52: 609-612, 1981.
203. Sasaki T, Ramamurthy NS, Golub LM. Tetracycline administration increases collagen synthesis in osteoblasts of streptozotocin-induced diabetic rats: A quantitative autoradiographic study. Calcif Tissue Int, 50: 411-419, 1992.
204. Greenwald RA, Simonson BG, Moak SA, Rush SW, Ramamurthy NS, Laskin RS, Golub LM. Inhibition of epiphyseal cartilage collagenase by tetracyclines in low phosphate rickets in rats. J Orthop Res, 6: 695-703, 1988.
205. Schlondorff D, Satriano J. Interactions with calmodulin: Potential mechanism for some inhibitory actions of tetracyclines and calcium channel blockers. Biochem Pharmacol, 34: 3391-3393, 1985.
206. Lauhio A, Salo T, Ding Y, Konttinen YT, Nordstrom D, Tschesche H, Lähdevirta J, Golub LM, Sorsa T. In vivo inhibition of human neutrophil collagenase (MMP-8) activity during long-term combination therapy of doxycycline and non-steriodal anti-inflammatory drugs (NSAID) in acute reactive arthritis. Clin Exp Immunol, 98: 21-28, 1994.
207. Lovejoy B, Cleasby A, Hassell AM, Longley K, Luther MA, Weigl D, McGeehan G, McElroy AB, Drewry D, Lambert MH. Structure of the catalytic domain of fibroblast collagenase complexed with an inhibitor. Science, 263: 375-377, 1994.
208. Uitto VJ, Firth JD, Nip L, Golub LM. Doxycycline and chemically modified tetracyclines inhibit gelatinase A (MMP-2) gene expression in human skin keratinocytes. Ann NY Acad Sci 732: 140-151, 1994.
209. van den Bogert C, Dontje BHJ, Holtrop M, Melis TE, Romijn JC, van Dongen JW, Kroon AM. Arrest of proliferation of renal and prostate carcinomas of human origin by inhibition of mitochondrial protein synthesis. Cancer Res, 46: 3283-3289, 1986.
210. Kroon AM, Dontje BHJ, Holtrop M, van den Bogert C. The mitochondrial genetic system as a target for chemotherapy: tetracyclines as cytostatics. Cancer Lett, 25: 33-40, 1984.
211. Sotomayor EA, Teicher BA, Schwartz GN, Holden SA, Menon K. Minocycline in combination with chemotherapy or radiation therapy in vitro and in vivo. Cancer Chemother Pharmacol, 30: 377-384, 1992.
212. Duivenvoorden WCM, Vukmirovic-Popovic S, Lhotàk S, Seidlitz E, Hirte HW, Tozer RG, Singh G. Doxycycline decreases tumor burden in a bone metastasis model of human breast cancer. Cancer Res, 62: 1588-1591, 2002.
213. Cianfrocca M, Cooley TP, Lee JY, Rudek MA, Scadden DT, Ratner L, Pluda JM, Figg WD, Krown SE, Dezube BJ. Matrix metalloproteinase inhibitor COL-3 in the treatment of AIDS-related Kaposi's sarcoma: a phase I AIDS malignancy consortium study. J Clin. Oncol, 20: 153-159, 2002.
214. Lin JT, Lane JM. Bisphosphonates. J Am Acad Orthop Surg, 11: 1-4, 2003.

215. Kanis JA, McCloskey EV. Bisphosphonates in multiple myeloma. Cancer, 88: 3022-3032, 2000.
216. Lipton A. Bisphosphonates and breast carcinoma. Cancer, 88: 3033-3037, 2000.
217. Eaton CL, Coleman RE. Pathophysiology of bone metastases from prostate cancer and the role of bisphosphonates in treatment. Cancer Treat Rev, 29: 189-198, 2003.
218. Paterson AHG, Powles TJ, McCloskey E, Hanson J, Ashley S. Double-blind controlled trial of clodronate in patients with bone metastases from breast cancer. J Clin Oncol, 11: 59-63, 1993.
219. O'Rourke N, McCloskey E, Houghton F, Huss H, Kanis JA. Double-blind, placebo controlled, dose-response trial of oral clodronate in patients with bone metastases. J Clin Oncol, 13: 929-934, 1995.
220. Kanis JA, Powles T, Paterson AHG, McCloskey EV, Ashley S. Clodronate decreases the frequency of skeletal metastases in women with breast cancer. Bone, 19: 663-667, 1996.
221. Diel IJ, Solomayer EF, Costa SD, Gollan C, Goerner R, Wallwiener D, Kaufmann M, Bastert G. Reduction in new metastases in breast cancer with adjuvant clodronate treatment. N Eng J Med, 339: 357-363, 1998.
222. Sasaki A, Boyce BF, Story B, Wright KR, Chapman M, Boyce R, Mundy GR, Yoneda, T. Bisphosphonate risedronate reduces metastatic human breast cancer burden in bone in nude mice. Cancer Res, 55: 3551-3557, 1995.
223. Stearns M, Wang M. Effects of alendronate and taxol on PC-3 ML cell bone metastases in SCID mice. Invasion Metastasis, 16: 116-131, 1996.

Chapter 13

THE ROLE OF BISPHOSPHONATES IN BONE METASTASIS

Mary MacKenzie and Pierre Major
Juravinski Cancer Centre, Hamilton, Ontario, Canada

1. INTRODUCTION

Bisphosphonates are analogs of pyrophosphate, which is a naturally occurring regulator of bone mineralization with the chemical structure P-O-P (see Figure 1). These compounds were first synthesized in Germany in 1865. Their initial use was industrial (textile, fertilizer and oil industries) and for prevention of mineral scaling (due to their ability to inhibit calcium carbonate precipitation). The biological properties of these compounds, however, were not explored until the 1960's (1, 2).

In the decades since their first clinical use, bisphosphonates have become an important tool in the treatment of a broad spectrum of diseases including Paget's disease, osteoporosis, and cancer. The role of bisphosphonates in the treatment of malignant disease is expanding. These agents have been successfully used in the treatment of bone metastases and malignancy-associated hypercalcemia; and their benefit in the adjuvant setting is being evaluated.

Bisphosphonates exert their effects through a variety of mechanisms. Their molecular mechanism of action, as well as their effects on osteoclasts, osteoblasts and tumor cells will be reviewed here.

G. Singh and W. Orr (eds.), Bone Metastasis and Molecular Mechanisms, 277-301.

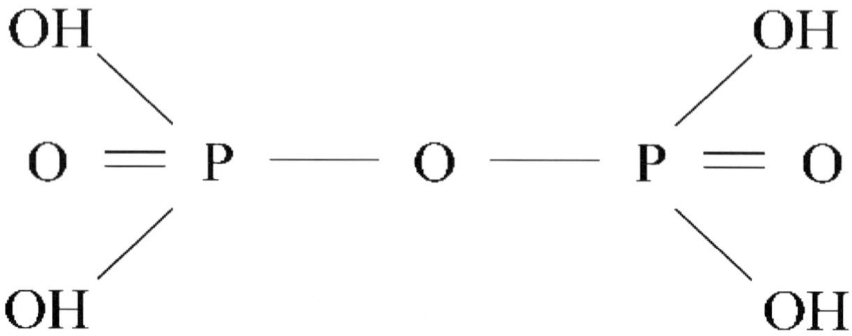

Figure 1. Pyrophosphate

2. MOLECULAR MECHANISMS OF ACTION

In bisphosphonates, carbon has replaced the central oxygen of the pyrophosphate structure. First generation bisphosphonates include clodronate and etidronate. Newer generation bisphosphonates (pamidronate, alendronate, ibandronate, risedronate and zoledronic acid) have a side chain containing one or more nitrogen atoms (see Figure 2). All bisphosphonates form a 3D structure capable of binding divalent ions including calcium. The affinity for calcium can be increased further if one of the side chains is a hydroxyl or a primary amino group (as with second generation bisphosphonates) because this allows the formation of a tridentate configuration that is able to bind to calcium more avidly (3).

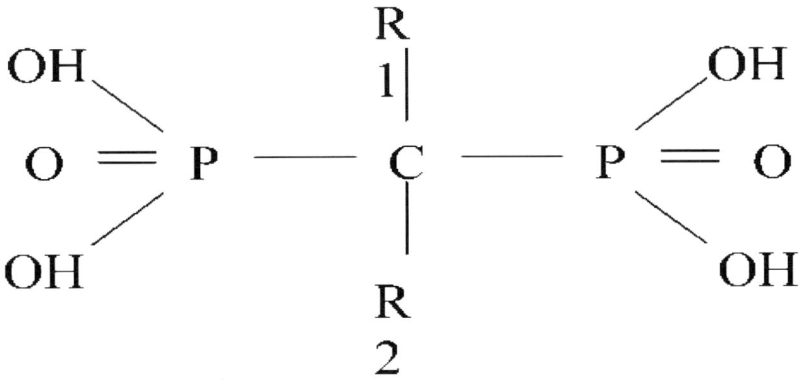

Figure2. Bisphosphonate

In both tumor cells and osteoclasts, first generation bisphophonates act through the formation of cytotoxic ATP-analogues after internalization by cells. These metabolites accumulate in the intracellular space and inhibit crucial ATP-dependant enzymes (4).

Newer, nitrogen-containing bisphosphonates exert their effect by inhibition of the mevalonate pathway (Figure 3). One enzyme that is specifically inhibited in this pathway is farnesyl diphosphate synthase (5). Inhibition of this enzyme results in a decrease in prenylation (post-translational modification) of small GTP-binding proteins that are essential for normal cell function. Such GTP-binding proteins include ras, rac and rho. Senaratne et al. (6) have shown that, in two lines of breast cancer cells, zoledronic acid impaired membrane localization of ras. This would indicate that prenylation (in this case, farnesylation) of this protein is reduced by the presence of this bisphosphonate. Likewise, Bergstrom et al. (7) also identified farnesyl diphosphate synthase as the selective target of alendronate in the mevalonate pathway.

This effect of nitrogen-containing bisphosphonates is not, however, limited to farnesylation. Coxon et al. (8) found that the inhibitory effect of nitrogen-containing bisphosphonates on bone resorption more likely results from the loss of a different set of prenylated proteins; the geranylgeranylated proteins. In their assays, GGTI-298 (a specific inhibitor of geranylgeranyl transferase I) prevented osteoclast formation in murine bone marrow cultures, inhibited bone resorption and promoted osteoclast apoptosis. In contrast to that finding, FTI-227 (a specific inhibitor of farnesyl transferase) had little effect on osteoclast apoptosis and did not inhibit bone resorption.

bisphosphonates subsequently cross the vacuolar membrane is not well understood.

3.1.1 Apoptosis of Osteoclasts

Both nitrogen and non-nitrogen-containing bisphosphonates result in osteoclast apoptosis. Hughes et al. (9) observed the effects of three bisphosphonates (risedronate, pamidronate and clodronate) on osteoclast survival. *In vitro* treatment of osteoclasts with bisphosphonates was again associated with 4- to 24-fold increase in the proportion of osteoclasts with apoptotic changes. This observation was repeated in normal mice, mice with increased bone resorption and mice with osteolytic metastases. Other authors have noted that in addition to these apoptotic changes, osteoclast actin-rings are disrupted (10).

Building on these observations, Ito et al. (11) observed the effects of a third generation bisphosphonate (incadronate) on the femur and tibia of rats. Apoptosis was identified in osteoclasts on the basis of characteristic changes in cell and nuclear morphology, including pyknotic nuclei with condensation and margination of heterochromatins and DNA fragmentation. These investigators also noted enlargement and fusion of nuclear envelopes, leading to leakage of nuclear contents into the cytoplasm in the late stages of apoptosis. Degradation of cellular organelles, including the Golgi apparatus, was seen.

This process of bisphosphonate-induced osteoclast apoptosis entails the activation of caspases. Caspases are a group of cysteine proteases that cleaves intracellular substrates including poly-adenosine diphosphate, protein kinase C, and nuclear lamin proteins. The major osteoclast protease activated by bisphosphonate treatment is caspase-3-like protease. This protease, which specifically cleaves peptides with the amino acid sequence asp-glu-val-asp, thus plays an important role in osteoclast apoptosis (4).

Selander et al. (12) studied the effects of clodronate and pamidronate on both osteoclasts and macrophages (which are ontogenetically related to osteoclasts). The investigators assessed the effects of several inhibitors of the apoptotic cascade in preventing clodronate-induced programmed cell death. None of the inhibitors tested could completely prevent clondronate-induced apoptosis. Partial protection was seen with staurosporine and homocysteine, suggesting that cytoplasmic protein kinase C-activated mechanisms play a role in clodronate-induced osteoclast apoptosis.

Other investigators have raised the question of whether osteoclast apoptosis is an absolutely necessary step in the process of bisphosphonate-induced inhibition of bone resorption. Halasy-Nagy et al. (13) studied the effects of both nitrogen-containing (alendronate and risedronate) and non-nitrogen-containing (clodronate and etidronate) bisphosphonates on osteoclasts *in vitro*. The investigators showed that the anti-apoptotic cascade inhibitor Z-VAD-FNK did not prevent inhibition of resorption of bone seen with nitrogen-containing bisphosphonates. In contrast to this finding, Z-VAD-FMK did block clodronate- and etidronate-mediated inhibition of bone resorption. This data suggests that induction of apoptosis plays a major role in etidronate and clodronate-mediated inhibition of resorption, but alendronate and risedronate suppression of resorption is independent of their effects on apoptosis.

Other experimental findings have also supported this assertion that osteoclast apoptosis is not always required in order to see inhibition of bone resorption. These studies show that inhibition of bone resorption by nitrogen-containing bisphosphonates was not associated with a decrease in osteoclast numbers except at very high concentrations. Hence, as well as causing osteoclast cell death, bisphosphonates can cause more subtle changes in osteoclast function that affect their ability to resorb bone (3).

3.1.2 Osteoclast Ruffled Borders

After osteoclasts adhere to bone surface, they exhibit features of highly polarized cytoplasmic organization, including ruffled borders (this border is the tortuous area of osteoclast plasma membrane that lies adjacent to the bone surface, and is essential for bone resorption) and clear zones (14). The clear zone surrounds the ruffled border and seals the extra-cellular resorbing compartment in which bone resorption takes place. Osteoclasts adhere to the bone surfaced though structures in the clear zones called podosomes. These podosomes consist of dots containing F-actin.

One consistent feature of osteoclasts treated with bisphosphonates (*in vitro* or *in vivo*) is the lack of this ruffled border. Early on in the clinical development of bisphosphonates, Miller and Jee (15) studied the electron microscopic features of the bones of growing rats following administration of the bisphosphonate C12MDP. The ruffled borders were generally less extensive than in control rats. Similarly, Sato et al. (16) demonstrated that osteoclasts from adult rats, when treated with alendronate, lost their ruffled border but the clear zone remained intact.

The effects of tiludronate on osteoclast morphology have been studied in mouse culture systems (14). The results of this experiment showed that tiludronate is selectively incorporated into polarized osteoclasts that have a ruffled border (i.e., those osteoclasts that are functioning). Similarly, Ito et al. (11) examined the cytochemical and ultrastructural features of osteoclasts after treatment with a third generation bisphosphonate. These osteoclasts became devoid of ruffled borders and detached from bone surface.

The same authours (17) also examined the effects of 3rd generation bisphosphonate on osteoclasts in osteosclerotic mice (*oc/oc* mice). In such mice, osteoclasts are small and devoid of ruffled borders. Therefore, bone resorption is reduced. In these mice, after treatment with bisphosphonates, the osteoclasts detached from the bone surface and became apoptotic. This evidence indicates that osteoclasts that lack ruffled borders are nevertheless still affected by bisphosphonates. Therefore, these cells must absorb the bisphosphonates from a site other than the ruffled borders.

Finally, Alakangas et al. (18) treated rat osteoclasts with alendronate. In this experiment, widening of sealing zone areas, incomplete organization of tight attachments and ruffled borders were observed. Osteoclasts appeared partially detached from bone surface (by contrast, clodronate bone surfaces were thoroughly resorbed). The authors concluded that, following treatment with alendronate, osteoclasts are inactivated by mechanisms that impair vesicle transport, and apoptosis is only a secondary phenomenon.

3.1.3 Effects on Osteoclastogenesis

Osteoclasts derive from precursor cells of macrophagic/monocyte lineage. These cells express receptor activator of NF-kappaB (RANK), which is a member of the tumour necrosis factor receptor superfamily. Following activation of RANK by its ligand, RANKL, differentiation, proliferation and survival of proteoclasts is promoted. RANKL is largely produced by cells of osteoblast lineage. It can also be secreted by immune cells and by some tumour cells. RANKL is, physiologically, kept in check by osteoprotegerin (OPG). OPG serves as a soluble decoy receptor, which blocks RANKL and thus prevents bone resorption. This normal balance between RANKL and OPG regulates the physiologic process of bone resorption and remodelling. When, however, this balance is disrupted by malignant tumours, skeletal complications of cancer ensue (19).

The effects of bisphosphonates on osteoclastogenesis in fetal rat calvariae have been studied by Evans et al. (20). All bisphosphonates tested were able to inhibit osteoclast formation at low concentrations. Little or no effect on osteoblasts was seen. Evidence also indicates that, in order for bisphosphonates to exert their anti-osteoclastogenic effects, they must be bound to bone mineral (21).

In an effort to elucidate the mechanism of this inhibition of osteoclastogenesis, Nishikawa et al. (22) examined the effects of the bisphosphonate YM175 on osteoclast-like multinucleated cell formation in cell culture. When osteoclast precursors of different tissue origins were treated with YM175, and co-cultured with calvarial osteoblasts, inhibition of osteoclast-like multinucleated cells was observed. When these osteoclast precursors were co-cultured with supporting cells of different origins (i.e. not osteoblasts), the results of treatment with YM175 varied. These findings suggest that YM175 inhibits osteoclastogenesis through its action on supporting cells of osteoblast lineage, rather than acting directly on the osteoclast precursors.

Clohisy et al. (23) used osteopetrotic (osteoclast-deficient) mice as an animal model to study the effect of pamidronate on a sarcoma that induces osteoclastogenesis. Experiments with this animal model suggested that pamidronate decreases the number of osteoclasts through its effects on myeloid precursor cells.

A separate mechanism of osteoclastogenesis inhibition is through increased production of osteoprotegerin from osteoblasts. A recent study confirmed that both pamidronate and zoledronic acid result in increased osteoprotegerin mRNA levels and OPG secretion in human osteoblasts (24).

In contrast to the above evidence, some investigators have found that bisphosphonates do not affect osteoclast formation. Breuil et al. (25) found that formation of osteoclast-like multinucleated cells from peripheral blood mononuclear cells was not inhibited by alendronate. Despite this data, the majority of studies support the hypothesis that some of the anti-resorptive activity of bisphosphonates is due to inhibition of osteoclastogenesis.

3.2 Effects on Osteoblasts

Reinholz et al. (26) studied the direct effects of bisphosphonates on cell proliferation, gene expression and bone formation in cultured fetal osteoblasts. Osteoblast cell proliferation was decreased, and cytodifferentiation was increased after treatment with pamidronate. These same authors, in a later study (27), found that zoledronic acid also induces human osteoblast differentiation via inhibition of the mevalonate pathway (i.e., the same pathway that is inhibited in osteoclasts). These *in vitro* observations, however, are probably not of physiologic significance, as is it known that bisphosphonates do not inhibit bone formation on a clinically important level (3).

Vitte et al. (28) studied the effect of ibandronate and alendronate on an osteoblastic cell line. When osteoclasts were cultured in medium that was taken from bisphosphonate-treated osteoblasts, pit formation (a measure of resorptive activity) was reduced by 50%. This suggests that the osteoblasts, when treated with bisphosphonates, secrete a soluble factor that inhibits osteoclast activity (later identified as osteoprotegerin). This hypothesis is supported by similar experiments by Yu et al. (29).

Alendronate has also been found to disrupt the modulatory effect of 1,25-dihydroxyvitamin D3 (a physiologic regulator of bone resorption) on parathyroid hormone-related peptide (PTHrP) production in human osteoblast cells. PHTrP is produced by several tumour types, and acts on PTH receptors to cause increased bone resorption. An increase in calcium influx appears to be involved in the mechanism mediating this effect of alendronate (30).

4. EFFECTS ON TUMOR CELLS

Many patients with malignant disease will eventually develop bone metastases. The incidence of bone involvement varies with the tumor type; in some diseases (multiple myeloma, breast and prostate cancer) the probability of bone metastases occurring is in excess of 65%. Bisphosphonates, through their effects on tumor adhesion, invasion, proliferation and on angiogenesis (in addition to their effects on bone), may have the potential to influence the clinical course of skeletal metastases.

4.1 Tumor Adhesion to Bone

Bisphosphonates strongly inhibit the binding of many human tumor cell line types, including breast and prostate, to bone. This effect has been seen regardless of whether the bone or the tumor cells were treated. Clezardin et al. (31) found that nitrogen-containing bisphosphonates inhibit tumor cell adhesion in a dose-dependant manner. The mechanism by which nitrogen-containing bisphosphonates inhibit tumor cell adhesion remains poorly understood. It is likely that modulation of cell adhesion molecules including cadherin, laminin and the integrins is involved.

Tumor adhesion to bone is a crucial step in the metastatic process. van der Pluijm et al. (32) used two *in vitro* models of bone matrix (cortical bone slices and cryostat sections of trabecular bone from neonatal mouse tails) to study the effects of bisphosphonate treatment on tumor adhesion. With these models, it was shown that four bisphosphonates (pamidronate, olpadronate, alendronate and ibandronate) inhibited adhesion and spreading of breast cancer cells in a dose-dependant manner.

The effect of bisphosphonates on breast and prostate carcinoma cell adhesion to unmineralized and mineralized bone extracellular matrices has been studied (33). Bisphosphonate pre-treatment of tumor cells inhibited tumor cell adhesion to unmineralized and mineralized osteoblastic extracellular membranes in a dose-dependant manner. They did not, in contrast, affect adhesion of normal cells (fibroblasts) to extracellular membranes.

4.2 Tumor Cell Invasion/ Matrix Metalloproteinases

Matrix metalloproteinases (MMPs) are a group of zinc-dependant endopeptidases involved in tissue remodeling (34). They are crucial to the ability of tumor cells to invade and metastasize, and are important in the maintenance and growth of metastatic foci. Nitrogen-containing bisphosphonates inhibit several MMPs. This inhibition is reversible with the addition of zinc, suggesting that the ability of bisphosphonates to chelate divalent ions is the mechanism by which they inhibit MMPs.

Teronen et al. (35) confirmed that the function of various MMP's is inhibited *in vitro* by bisphosphonates. In enzyme activity tests using purified and recombinant enzymes, they observed that the inhibition of MMP-1,2,3,7,8,9,12,13,14 activity by clodronate, alendronate, zoledronic acid, and nedrinate. Clodronate downregulates the expression of MT1-MMP protein and mRNA in several cell lines. Also, several bisphosphonates decreased the invasion of melanoma and fibrosarcoma cell lines through the artificial basement membrane, Matrigel.

Clodronate also inhibits MMP-8-mediated degradation of casein and type 1 collagen, and has inhibitory effects on MMP-9 and –2. The nitrogen-containing bisphosphonates pamidronate and alendronate inhibits activity of MMP-3. Zoledronic acid has been shown to inhibit MMP-3.

Derenne et al. (36) found that zoledronic acid inhibits the production of MMP-1 (the major MMP involved in the initiation of bone metastases) by bone marrow stromal cells. Similarly, Ichinose et al. (37) investigated the role of bisphosphonates in the production of MMP-2 from human osteoblasts. Production was reduced in the presence of physiologic levels of plasmin.

However, conflicting data prevents the drawing of firm conclusions. For example zoledronic acid did not cause decreased expression of MMP-2 and -9 from breast cancer cells (33).

4.3 Tumor Cell Proliferation and Survival

An inhibitory effect of bisphosphonates on the growth of myeloma, melanoma, breast and prostate cancer cell lines has been observed (31). Concentrations of 10^{-5} to 10^{-4} are required to inhibit cellular proliferation. These concentrations are significantly higher than would be present in serum. However, they may be reached in bone at sites of active resorption, given that bisphosphonates avidly adhere to bone. As is true for osteoclasts, the major mechanism responsible for tumor cell apoptosis appears to be caspase activation (38).

4.5 Effects on Angiogenesis

Angiogenesis (the formation of new, tumour-associated, blood vessels) is essential for the establishment and growth of primary tumors and metastases. There is abundant evidence that bisphosphonates inhibit this process.

Zoledronic acid has been proven *in vitro* to inhibit the proliferation of human umbilical vein endothelial cells (an assay of antiangiogenic activity) normally induced by basic fibroblast growth factor, vascular endothelial growth factor and serum. When administered systemically to mice, zoledronic acid also potently inhibits the angiogenesis induced by subcutaneous implants impregnated with basic fibroblast growth factor (40).

A tissue model of angiogenesis has been developed using the prostates of castrated rats, in which the effects of bisphosphonates on testosterone-induced revascularization could be studied. Ibandronate and zoledronate, when given in combination with testosterone, induced a 50% reduction of revascularization in tests of blood vessel immunostaining (41).

Croucher et al. (42) investigated the effect of zoledronic acid on the development of bone disease, tumor burden and disease free survival on the 5T2MM model of multiple myeloma. Myeloma cells were injected intravenously into mice. The animals were then treated with zoledronic acid. Treatment was associated with a reduction in tumor burden and reduced angiogenesis as measured by microvessel density in myelomatous bone lesions.

Zoledronic acid modulates the endothelial cell surface receptors involved in angiogenesis. Such receptors, including alpha vBeta3 and alpha vBeta5 integrins and the 65kD laminin receptor, were downregulated on human endothelial cells after treatment with zoledronic acid (38).

In terms of clinical evidence for inhibition of angiogenesis, Santini et al. (43) evaluated the modification of angiogenetic cytokines after pamidronate infusion in 25 cancer patients with bone metastases. Basic Vascular Endothelial Growth Factor (which has been cited as a possible surrogate marker for angiogenic activity) levels decreased significantly at 1, 2 and 7 days after pamidronate treatment.

4.6 Synergism with Chemotherapy

As the use of bisphosphonates in the treatment of bone metastases increases, more patients will be receiving such treatment in combination with palliative chemotherapy. The evidence relating to the possible synergistic effects of bisphosphonates and chemotherapy is discussed below.

The anti-tumor effects of several chemotherapeutic agents are potentiated by bisphosphonates. Clezardin et al. (31) has studied the effects of combined ibandronate and taxanes in breast cancer cell lines. Inhibitory effects on adhesion and invasion of bone were observed. Also, zoledronic acid combined with paclitaxel exerts a synergistic proapoptotic effect on breast cancer cell lines (44). In murine models of bone metastases from breast carcinoma cells, the combination of ibandronate and doxorubicin suppressed bone (and visceral) metastases more effectively than either agent alone (45).

Zoledronic acid has also shown an additive effect when combined with the COX-2 inhibitor SC236. Witters et al. (46) observed that zoledronic acid alone caused a 23% reduction in growth of prostate cancer cells, while SC236 caused a 40% reduction. When these agents were combined, a 60% reduction in tumor growth was observed.

5. CLINICAL USE OF BISPHOSPHONATES IN CANCER PATIENTS

Skeletal metastases are a common problem, particularly with cancer of the breast, prostate, lung and with multiple myeloma. Complications of skeletal metastases include bone pain, pathologic fractures, hypercalcemia and spinal cord compression. Several treatment modalities are available for the treatment of bone pain, including radiotherapy, analgesics and bisphosphonates. Prior to the era of bisphosphonates, hypercalcemia was treated acutely with volume expansion, calcitonin, plicamycin, and loop diuretics. These agents were of limited efficacy, and today, bisphosphonates are considered to be standard management in the care of such patients.

5.1 Breast Cancer

At least 25% of women diagnosed with breast cancer will eventually develop bone metastases. On average, these patients will have a complication (such as pain and fracture) from their bone metastases once every three to four months (47).

Several large multicentre trials have examined the effects of bisphosphonates in the treatment of both early and advanced breast cancer (see Table 1). A systematic review of randomized trials has been performed (48). In eight studies that included 1962 women with advanced breast cancer and existing bone metastases, bisphosphonates reduced the risk of developing a skeletal event by 14% (relative risk 0.86, 95% confidence interval 0.8-0.91;$p<0.00001$). All studies of intravenous pamidronate and oral clodronate in women with advanced breast cancer and bone metastases showed significant delays in median time to a skeletal event.

Bisphosphonates are also associated with a reduction in bone pain; compared with placebo or no treatment, bisphosphonates significantly improved pain scores in four trials. Treatment with bisphosphonates does not; however, appear to affect survival in women with advanced breast cancer.

Table 1. Clinical Trials of Bisphosphonates in Breast Cancer Patients

Trial	Compound /Dose	Patients	Endpoints	Outcome	Comments
Paterson et al., 1993[55]	Clodronate 1600 mg/day	173	HCM, radiotherapy, fractures	Fewer vertebral fractures and less HCM, no difference in complications	104 patients died prior to 18 month follow-up
Kanis et al., 1996[56]	Clodronate 1600 mg/day	133	Development of bone mets and related clinical events	Fewer bone mets and clinical events; no difference in proportion of affected patients	Prevention study
Hortobagyi et al., 1996[57]	Pamidronate 90 mg IV vs. placebo	382	Median time to SRE; proportion of patients with SRE	Time to SRE:1.31m vs. 7 m (favor pamidronate);43 % with SRE for pamidronate. vs. 56%	
Diel et al., 1998[49]	Clodronate 1600 mg/day	302	Incidence and extent of new metastases	Lower incidence of osseous and visceral mets in the treatment group	Prevention study in patients with tumor cells in bone marrow
Kristensen et al., 1999[58]	Clodronate 1600 mg/day	100	Skeletal events including HCM, fractures and radiotherapy	Temporary reduction in number of skeletal events in treatment group	No effect on disease progression in bone or survival
Theriault et al., 1999[59]	Pamidronate 90 mg IV vs. placebo	372	Median time to SRE; proportion of patients with SRE	10.4 vs. 6.9 mos. (favor pamidronate); 56% pamidronate with SRE compared to 67% placebo	treatment X 28 weeks; more vomiting leukopenia with pamidronate than placebo
Saarto et al., 2001[50]	Clodronate 1600 mg/day daily vs. control	299	Incidence bone mets, nonosseous mets, OS, DFS	No difference in bone mets (21% vs. 17%); more nonosseous mets in clodronate	Prevention trial, patients received adjuvant chemotherapy and hormonal

Trial	Compound /Dose	Patients	Endpoints	Outcome	Comments
				group (43% vs, 25%); OS and DFS lower in clodronate group	therapy
Rosen et al., 2001[60]	Zoledronic acid 4 mg vs. 8 mg IV vs. Pamidronate 90 mg IV	1648	SRE	No difference in proportion with SRE's on zoledronic acid decreased incidence of bone radiation	Patients with skeletal mets from breast cancer or osteolytic myeloma
Powles et al., 2002[61]	Clodronate 1600 mg/day vs. placebo	1069	Relapse in bone and other sites, mortality, toxicity	Sig. reduction in bone mets during treatment period only; no difference in visceral mets. Sig. reduction in mortality	Prevention trial

HCM: hypercalcemia
SRE: Skeletal Related Events
OS: Overall survival
DFS: Disease free survival

The data regarding the use of bisphosphonates in early breast cancer is less compelling. In three studies of oral clodronate that included 1680 women with early breast cancer, there was borderline evidence of a reduction in the risk of developing skeletal metastases (RR 0.73, 95% CI 0.55-0.98;p=0.04). It should be noted that the populations of these trials were quite heterogeneous. Diel's trial of oral clodronate in 302 early breast cancer patients who were felt to be at high risk for recurrence (on the basis of bone marrow micrometastastases) showed a lower incidence of bone metastases, and surprisingly, a lower incidence of visceral metastases in the clodronate group (49). This study was, however, refuted by Saarto's trial of 299 patients with node-positive operable breast cancer; here, bone metastases were detected with equal frequency in both the treatment and control groups (50). Interestingly, there was a *higher* incidence of non-osseous metastases and *lower* overall survival in the treatment group.

5.2 Multiple Myeloma

Multiple myeloma is a neoplastic disorder of plasma cells, and accounts for 10% of all haematologic malignancies. The mechanism of bone destruction in myeloma is a result of both increased osteoclast and decreased osteoblast activity. These bone changes frequently lead to lytic lesions, particularly within the vertebral column. Hypercalcemia also will develop in 25% of patients with myeloma (51). For these reasons, bisphosphonates are increasingly being used in the management of this disease (see Table 2).

Table 2. Clinical Trials of Bisphosphonates in Multiple Myeloma Patients

Trial	Compound/ Dose	Patients	Endpoints	Outcome	Comments
Belch et al., 1991[62]	Etidronate 5/mg/kg/day	173	Height, HCM, path fractures, bone pain	No difference from placebo for any measure	Higher dose of 20mg/kg/day discontinued
Lahtinen et al., 1992[63]	Clodronate 2400mg/day	336	Osteolytic progression	Less progression with clodronate	No effect on fractures, bone pain or HCM
Brincker et al., 1998[64]	oral pamidronate 300 mg/day	300	Skeletal complications	No difference from placebo for skeletal-related morbidity	No influence on survival or hypercalcemia. Less pain in treatment group
Berenson et al., 1998[65]	Pamidronate 90 mg intravenously	392	SRE	Trend to lower SRE rate in treatment group (p=0.15)	No survival benefit
Terpos et al., 2000[66]	Pamidronate 90 mg intravenously	62	SRE	No changes in SRE's	Given synchronously with chemotherapy, pamidronate reduces markers of bone turnover
McCloskey et al., 2001[67]	Clodronate 1600 mg/day	619	Pathologic fracture, HCM, performance status, bone pain	Fewer fractures, no difference in HCM; survival benefit only in subgroup with no skeletal fractures at presentation	Follow up > 8 years
Rosen et al., 2001[60]	Zoledronic acid 4mg vs. 8 mg IV vs. Pamidronate 90mg iv	1648	SRE	No difference in proportion with SRE's on zoledronic acid decreased incidence of bone radiation	Patients with skeletal mets from breast cancer or osteolytic myeloma
Menssen et al., 2002[68]	intravenous ibandronate 2mg iv vs placebo		SRE	No difference in SRE's bone pain, median survival	Post hoc analyses showed suppression of bone turnover markers

A systematic review of trials related to the use of bisphosphonates in myeloma has been conducted (52). Eleven trials including 1113 patients were analysed. All were randomised trials comparing bisphosphonates to placebo or no treatment. The pooled analysis of these trials showed a beneficial effect of bisphosphonates in terms of the prevention of pathological vertebral fractures and improvement of pain (Odds Ratio 0.59; 95% CI 0.45-0.78; p=0.0001). There was no significant effect of bisphosphonates on mortality, reduction of non-vertebral fractures, or on the incidence of hypercalcemia.

5.3 Prostate Cancer

Please also see Table 3 for an overview of clinical trials of bisphosphonates in prostate cancer.

Excluding superficial skin cancers, prostate cancer is the most common malignancy afflicting North American men (51). This cancer has a strong propensity to metastasize to bone, often in the form of osteoblastic lesions. These metastases most commonly affect the pelvis, ribs, and spine. Those that affect the spine have the potential to cause postural changes, deformity, and, when they compress the spinal cord, significant neurologic impairment.

Several clinical trials have assessed the potential benefit of bisphosphonates in the management of prostate cancer patients with bone metastases. Many of the initial trials were statistically underpowered to detect any benefit in terms of pain or skeletal event rate. Most of these trials did not support the role of bisphosphonates in the treatment of prostate cancer-related bone pain.

A larger, more recent trial (53) has evaluated the role of zoledronic acid in prostate cancer patients. Two doses (8 and 4 mg) were compared to placebo. The 8mg arm was terminated prematurely due to concerns regarding renal toxicity. The trial showed a clinically significant advantage for zoledronic acid compared to placebo in terms of reduction of the proportion of patients any skeletal complication or pathologic fracture. Zoledronic acid also significantly reduced bone pain compared with placebo at 3 and 9 months.

Prostate cancer is often treated with androgen deprivation therapy, and this treatment has the potential to cause osteoporotic changes, thus compounding the deleterious bone effects of the disease itself. The role of clodronate in the prevention of osteopenia has been studied by Smith et al. (54) in patients with nonmetastatic prostate cancer who are receiving androgen deprivation therapy. Patients receiving clodronate had an increase in bone density of 5.6%. Those receiving placebo had a mean decrease in bone density of 2.2%. Although this evidence is preliminary, it would support the use of clodronate in this setting.

Table 3. Clinical Trial of Bisphosphonates in Prostate Cancer Patients

Trial	Compound/ Dose	Patients	Endpoints	Outcome	Comments
Smith et al., 1989[69]	Etidronate 7.5 mg/kg IV for 3 days then 400 mg/day oral	57	Bone pain, skeletal lesions	No difference from placebo	Four treatment groups
Strang et al., 1997[70]	Clodronate intravenously followed by orally 1600mg/day vs. placebo	55	Pain assessment with visual analog scale	No difference in pain	Trial ended prematurely due to poor recruitment
Pelger et al., 1998[71]	Olpadronate 4 mg intravenously	28	Biochemical and clinical response	Decrease in urinary hydroxyproline excretion; decrease in bone pain in 75% patient	Trial not statistically powered to detect clinical benefit
Heidenreich et al., 2001[72]	Clodronate IV 300 mg for 8 days then 1600 mg daily	85	Pain and analgesia use, performance status and mobility	Decrease in pain and performance status	Nonrandomized study
Heidenreich et al., 2002[73]	Ibandronate 6 mg intravenously	25	Pain reduction using visual analog scale	Significant reduction in pain score in 92%, 39% pain free	Increase in Karnofsky index paralleled decrease pain
Saad et al., 2002[53]	Zoledronic acid 4mg vs. 8 mg vs. placebo	643	Skeletal related events (SRE), time to first SRE, pain	Reduction in proportion of patients with SRE's, non-significant reduction in time to SRE's, reduction in pain	Renal toxicity with zoledronic acid 8 mg, therefore, discontinued
Ernst et al., 2002[7]	Mitoxantrone+ prednisone+ clodronate vs. Mitoxantrone+ prednisone alone	208	Assessment of quality of life and health resource utilization	Non-significant decrease in pain	Multicentre trial

Trial	Compound/ Dose	Patients	Endpoints	Outcome	Comments
Smith et al., 2003[54]	Zoledronic acid 4 mg vs. placebo	106	Percent change (from baseline to 1 year) in bone mineral density of the lumbar spine	Mean bone density increased by 5.6% in treatment arm, decreased by 2.2% in controls	Trial in patients with nonmetastatic prostate cancer receiving androgen deprivation therapy

ACKNOWLEDGEMENTS

We wish to thank Dr. G. Singh for his kind assistance with this chapter, and also E. Seidlitz for his assistance with the illustrative figures.

REFERENCES

1. Fleisch H, Russel RG, Francis MD. Diphosphonates inhibit hydroxyapatite dissolution in vitro and bone absorption in tissue culture and in vivo. Science, 165:1262-1264, 1996.
2. Fliesch H. Bisphosphonates in Bone Disease: From the Laboratory to the Patient. Parthenon Publishing Group Inc. 1997.
3. Rogers MJ, Gordon S, Benford HL, Coxon FP, Luckman SP, Monkkonen J, Frith JC. Cellular and Molecular Mechanisms of Action of Bisphosphonates. Cancer, 88: 2961-2978, 2000.
4. Benford HL, McGowan NWA, Helfrich MH, Nuttall ME, Rogers MJ. Visualization of bisphosphonate-induced caspase-3 activity in apoptotic osteoclasts in vitro. Bone. 28: 65-473, 2001.
5. Dunford JE, Thompson K, Coxon FP, Luckman SP, Hahn FM, Poulter CD, Ebetineo FH, Rogers MJ. Structure-activity relationships for inhibition of farnesyl diphosphonate synthase in vitro and inhibition of bone resorption in vivo by nitrogen-containing bisphosphonates. J Pharmacol Exp Ther, 296: 235-242, 2001.
6. Senaratne SG, Colston KW. Direct effects of bisphosphonates on breast cancer cells. Breast Cancer Rev, 4: 18-23. 2002.
7. Bergstrom JD, Bostedor RG, Masarachia PJ, Reszka AA, Rodan G. Alendronate is a specific, nanomolar inhibitor of farnesyl disphosphonate synthase. Arch Biochem Biophys, 373: 231-241, 2000.
8. Coxon FP, Helfrich MH, Van't Hof R, Sebti S, Ralston SH, Hamilton A, Rogers MJ. Protein geranylgeranylation is required for osteoclast formation, function, and survival: inhibition by bisphosphonates and GGTI-298. J Bone Miner Res, 15: 1467-1476, 2000.
9. Hughes DE, Wright KR, Uy HL, Sasaki A, Yoneda T, Roodman GD, Mundy GR, Boyce BF. Bisphosphonates promote apoptosis in murine osteoclasts in vitro and in vivo. J Bone Miner Res, 10:1478-1487, 1995.

10. Hiroi-Furuya E, Kameda T, Hiura K, Mano H, Miyazawa K, Nakamaru Y, Watanabe-Mano M, Okuda N, Shimada J, Yamamoto Y, Hakdea Y, Kumegawa M. Etidronate (EHDP) inhibits osteoclastic-bone resorption, promotes apoptosis and disrupts actin rings in isolate-mature osteoclasts. Calcif Tissue Int, 64: 219-223, 1999.
11. Ito M, Amizuka N, Nakajima T, Ozawa H. Ultrastructural and cytochemical studies on cell death of osteoclasts induced by bisphosphonate treatment. Bone, 25: 447-452, 1999.
12. Selander KS, Monkkonen J, Karhukorpi EK, Harkonen P, Hannuniemi R, Vaananen HK. Characteristics of clodronate-induced apoptosis in osteoclasts and macrophages. Mol Pharmacol, 50: 1127-1138, 1996.
13. Halasy-Nagy JM, Rodan GA, Reska AA. Inhibition of bone resorption by alendronate and risedronate does not require osteoclast apoptosis. Bone, 29: 553-559, 2001.
14. Murakami H, Takahashi N, Sasaki T, Udagawa N, Tanaka S, Nakamura I, Zhang D, Barbier A, Suda A. A possible mechanism of the specific action of bisphosphonates on osteoclasts: tiludronate preferentially affects polarized osteoclasts having ruffled borders. Bone, 17: 137-144, 1995.
15. Miller SC, Jee WS. The effect of dichloromethylene diphosphonate, a pyrophosphate analog, on bone and bone cell structure in the growing rat. Anat Rec, 193: 439-462, 1979.
16. Sato M, Grasser W, Endo N, Akins R, Simmons H, Thompson DD, Golub E, Rodan GA. Bisphosphonate action. Alendronate localization in rat bone and effects on osteoclast ultrastructure. Clin Invest, 88: 2095-2105, 1991.
17. Ito M, Amizuka N, Nakajima T, Ozawa H. Bisphosphonate acts on osteoclasts independent of ruffled borders in osteosclerotic (oc/oc) mice. Bone, 28: 609-616, 2001.
18. Alakangas A, Selander K, Mulari M, Helleen J, Lehenkari P, Monkkonen J, Salo J, Vaanenen K. Alendronate disturbs vesicular trafficking in osteoclasts. Calcif Tissue, 70: 40-47, 2002.
19. Sezar O, Heider U, Zavrski I, Kuhne CA, Hofbauer LC. RANK ligand and osteoprotegerin in myeloma bone disease. Blood, 10: 2094-2098, 2003.
20. Evans CE, Braidman IP. Effects of two novel bisphosphonates on bone cells in vitro. Bone Miner, 26: 95-107, 1994.
21. Lowik CW, van der Pluijm G, van der Wee-Pals LJ, Van Treslong-De Groot HB, Bijvoet OL. Migration and phenotypic transformation of osteoclast precursors into mature osteoclasts: the effect of a bisphosphonate. Bone Miner Res, 3: 185-192, 1998.
22. Nishikawa M, Yamamoto M, Murakami T, Akatsu T, Kugai N, Nagata N. A third-generation bisphosphonate, YM175, inhibits osteoclast formation in murine cocultures by inhibiting proliferation of precursor cells via support cell-dependent mechanisms. J Bone Miner Res, 13: 986-995, 1998.
23. Clohisy DR, O'Keefe PF, Ramnaraine ML. Pamidronate decreases tumor-induced osteoclastogenesis in osteopetrotic mice. J Orthop Res, 19: 554-558, 2001.
24. Viereck V, Emons G, Lauck V. Bisphosphonates pamidronate and zoledronic acid stimulate osteoprotegerin production by primary human osteoblasts. Biochem Res Commun, 291: 680-686, 2002.
25. Breuil V, Cosman F, Stein L, Hobart W, Nieves J, Shen V. Human osteoclast formation and activity in vitro: effects of alendronate. J Bone Miner Res, 13: 1721-1729, 1998.
26. Reinholz GG, Getz B, Pederson L, Sanders ES, Subramaniam M, Ingle JN, Spelsberg TC. Bisphosphonates directly regulate cell proliferation, differentiation, and gene expression in human osteoblasts. Cancer Res, 60:6001-6007, 2000.
27. Reinholz GG, Getz B, Sanders ES, Karpeisky MY, Padyukova NSh, Mikhailov SN, Ingle JN, Spelsberg TC. Distinct mechanisms of bisphosphonate action between

osteoblasts and breast cancer cells: identity of a potent new bisphosphonate analogue. Breast Cancer Res, 71: 257-268, 2002.
28. Vitte C, Fleisch H, Guenther HL. Bisphosphonates induce osteoblasts to secrete an inhibitor of osteoclast-mediated resorption. Endocrinology, 137: 2324-2333, 1996.
29. Yu X, Scholler J, Foged NT. Interaction between effects of parathyroid hormone and bisphosphonate on regulation of osteoclast activity by the osteoblast-like cell line UMR-106. Bone, 19: 339-345, 1996.
30. Gomez-Garcia L, Esbrit P, Carreno L, Sabando P, Garcia-Flores M, Martinez ME. Alendronate interacts with the inhibitory effect of 1,25(OH)2D3 on parathyroid hormone-related protein expression in human osteoblastic cells. J Bone Miner Res,18: 78-87, 2003.
31. Clezardin P, Fournier P, Boissier S, Peyruchaud O. In vitro and in vivo antitumor effects of bisphosphonates. Curr Med Chem, 10: 173-180, 2003.
32. van der Pluijm G, Vloedgraven H, van Beek E, van der Wee-Pals L, Lowik C, Papapoulos S. Bisphosphonates inhibit the adhesion of breast cancer cells to bone matrices in vitro. J Clin Invest, 98: 698-705, 1996.
33. Boissier S, Ferreras M, Payruchaud O, Magnetto S, Ebetino FH, Colombel M, Delmas P, Delaisse JM, Clezardin P. Bisphosphonates inhibit breast and prostate carcinoma cell invasion, an early event in the formation of bone metastases. Cancer Res, 60: 2949-2054, 2000.
34. Neville-Webbe HL, Holen I, Coleman RE. The anti-tumor activity of bisphosphonates. Cancer Treat Rev, 28: 305-319, 2000.
35. Teronen O, Heikkila P, Konttinen YT, Laitinen M, Salo T, Hanemaaijer R, Teronen A, Maisi P, Sorsa T. MMP inhibition and downreguation by bisphosphonates. Ann NY Acad Sci, 878: 453-465, 1999.
36. Derenne S, Amiot M, Barille S, Collette M, Robillard N, Berthaud P, Harousseau JL, Bataille R. Zoledronate is a potent inhibitor of myeloma cell growth and secretion of IL-6 and MMP-1 by the tumoral environment. J Bone Miner Res, 14: 2048-2056, 1999.
37. Ichinose Y, Migita K, Nakashima T, Kawakami A, Aoyagi T, Eguchi K. Effects of bisphosphonate on the release of MMP-2 from cultured human osteoblasts. Tohuko J Exp Med, 192: 111-118, 2000
38. Green J. Bisphosphonates in cancer therapy. Curr Opin Oncol, 14: 609-615, 2002.
39. Corey E, Brown LG, Quinn JE, Poot M, Roudier MP, Higano CS, Vessella RL. Zoledronic acid exhibits inhibitory effects on osteoblastic and osteolytic metastases of prostate cancer. Clin Cancer Res, 9: 295-306, 2003.
40. Wood J, Bonjean K, Ruetz S, Bellahcene A, Devy L, Foidart JM, Castronovo V, Green JR. Novel antiangiogenic effects of the bisphosphonate compound zoledronic acid. J Pharmacol Exp Ther, 302: 1055-1061, 2002.
41. Fournier P, Boissier S, Filleur S, Guglielmi J, Cabon F, Colombel M, Clezardin P. Bisphosphonates inhibit angiogenesis in vitro and testosterone-stimulated vascular regrowth in the ventral prostate in castrated rats. Cancer Res, 62: 6538-6544, 2002.
42. Croucher PI, De Hendrick R, Perry MJ, Hijzen A, Shipman CM, Lippitt J, Green J, Van Marck E, Van Camp B, Vanderkerken K. Zoledronic acid treatment of 5T2MM-bearing mice inhibits the development of myeloma bone disease: evidence for decreased osteolysis, tumor burden and angiogenesis, and increased survival. J Bone Miner Res, 18: 483-492, 2003.
43. Santini D, Vicenzi B, Avvisati G, Dicuonzo G, Battistoni F, Gavasci M. Salerno A, Denaro V, Tonini G. Pamidronate induces modifications of circulating angiogenetic factors in cancer patients. Clin Cancer Res; 8: 1080-1084, 2002.

44. Jagdev SP, Coleman RE, Shipman CM, Rostami A, Croucher PI. The bisphosphonate, zoledronic acid, induces apoptosis of breast cancer cells: evidence for synergy with paclitaxel. Br J Cancer; 84: 1126-1134, 2001.
45. Yoneda T, Michigami T, Yi B, Williams PJ, Niewlona M, Hiraga T. Actions of bisphosphonate on bone metastasis in animal models of breast carcinoma. Cancer, 88: 2979-2988, 2000.
46. Witters L, Crispino J, Javeed M. Inhibition of growth of a human prostate cancer cell line with the combination of zoledronic acid and a COX-2 inhibitor. (Abst) Proc Am Soc Clin Oncol, 1827, 2002.
47. Brown JE, Coleman RE. The present and future role of bisphosphonates in the management of patients with breast cancer. Breast Cancer Res, 4:24-29, 2002.
48. Pavlakis N, Stockler M. Bisphosphonates for breast cancer. Cochrane Database Syst Rev, (1):CD003474, 2002.
49. Diel I, Solomayer ER, Costa SD, Gollan C, Goener R. eduction in new metastases in breast cancer with adjuvant clodronate treatment. N Engl J Med, 339: 357-363, 1998.
50. Saarto T, Blomqvist C, Virkkunen P, Elomaa I. Adjuvant clodronate treatment dose not reduce the frequency of skeletal metastases in node-positive breast cancer patients: 5-year results of a randomized controlled trial. J Clin Oncol, 19: 10-17, 2001.
51. DeVita VT, Hellman S, Rosenburg S. Cancer: Principles and Practice of Oncology Sixth Edition. Lippincott, Williams and Wilkins 2002.
52. Djulbegovic B, Wheatly K, Ross J, Clark O, Bos G, Goldschmidt H, Cremer F, Alsina M, Glasmacher A. Bisphosphonates in multiple myeloma. The Cochrane Library 2002 .
53. Saad F, Gleason DM, Marray R, Tchekmedyian S, Venner P, Lacombe L, Chin JL, Vinholes JJ, Goas J, Chen B. A randomized, placebo-controlled trial of zoledronic acid in patients with hormone-refractory prostate carcinoma. J Natl Cancer Inst, 94: 1458-1468, 2002.
54. Smith MR, Eastham J, Gleason DM, Shasha D, Tchekmedyian S, Zinner N. Randomized controlled trial of zoledronic acid to prevent bone loss in men receiving androgen deprivation therapy for nonmetastatic prostate cancer. J Urol, 169: 2008-2012, 2003.
55. Paterson AHG, Powles TJ, Kanis JA. Double blind controlled trial of oral clodronate in patients with bone metastases from breast cancer. J Clin Oncol, 11: 59-65, 1993.
56. Kanis JA, Powles T, Paterson AHG. Clodronate decreases the frequency of skeletal metastases in women with breast cancer. Bone, 19: 663-667, 1996.
57. Hortobagyi GN, Theriault RL, Porter L, Blaney D, Lipton A, Sinoff C. Efficacy of pamidronate in reducing skeletal complications in patients with breast cancer and lytic bone metastases. N Engl J Med, 335: 1785-1791, 1996.
58. Kristensen B, Ejlertsen B, Groenvold M, Hein S, Loft H, Mouridsen HT. Oral clodronate in breast cancer patients with bone metastases: a randomised study. J Intern Med, 246: 67-74, 1999.
59. Theriault RL, Lipton A, Hortobagyi GN, Leff R, Gluck S, Stewart JF, Costello S, Kennedy I. Pamidronate reduces skeletal morbidity in women with advanced breast cancer and lytic bone lesions: A randomised placebo-controlled trial. J Clin Oncol, 17: 846-854, 1999.
60. Rosen LS, Gordon D, Kaminski M, Howell A, Belch A, Mackey JA Zoledronic acid versus pamidronate in the treatment of skeletal metastases in patients with breast cancer or osteolytic lesions of multiple myeloma: A phase III, double-blind, comparative trial. Cancer J, 7: 377-87, 2001.

61. Powles T, Paterson S, Kanis JA, McCloskey E, Ashley S, Tidy A. Randomised placebo-controlled trial of clodronate in patients with primary operable breast cancer. J Clin Oncol, 20: 3219-3224, 2002.
62. Belch AR, Bergsagel DE, Wilson K, O'Reilly S, Wilson J, Sutton D, Pater J, Johnston D, Zee B. Effect of daily etidronate on the osteolysis of multiple myeloma. J Clin Oncol, 9: 1397-1402, 1991.
63. Lahtinen R, Laasko M, Palva I, Virkkunen P, Elomaa I. Randomised, placebo-controlled multicentre trial of clodronate in multiple myeloma. Lancet, 340: 1049-1052, 1992.
64. Brinker H, Westin J, Abildgaard N, Gimsing P, Turesson I, Hedenus M, Ford J, Kandra A. Failure of oral pamidronate to reduce skeletal morbidity in multiple myeloma: a double-blind placebo-controlled trial. Br J Haematol, 101: 280-286, 1998.
65. Berenson JR, Lichtenstein A, Porter L, Dimopoulos MA, Bordoni R, George S, Lipton A, Keller A. Long term pamidronate treatment of advanced multiple myeloma patients reduces skeletal events. J Clin Oncol, 16: 593-602, 1998.
66. Terpos E, Palermos J, Tsionos K, Anargyrou K, Vinious N Effect of pamidronate administration on markers of bone turnover and disease activity in multiple myeloma. Eur J Haematol, 65: 331-336, 2000.
67. Mccloskey EV, Dunn JA, Kanis JA, MacLennan IC, Drayson MT. Long-term follow-up of a prospective, double-blind, placebo-controlled randomised trial of clodronate in multiple myeloma. Br J Haematol, 113: 1035-43, 2001.
68. Menssen HD, Sakalova A, Fontana A, Herrmann Z, Boewer C, Facon T, Lichinitser MR, Singer CR. Effects of long-term intravenous ibandronate therapy on skeletal-related events, survival, and bone resorption markers in patients with advanced multiple myeloma. J Clin Oncol, 20: 2353-2359, 2002.
69. Smith JA. Palliation of painful bone metastases from prostate cancer using sodium etidronate: results of a randomized, prospective, double-blind, placebo-controlled study. J Urol, 141: 85-87, 1989.
70. Strang P, Nilsson S, Brandstedt S, Sehlin J, Borghede G, Varenhorst E, Bandman U, Borck L, EnglundG, Selin L. The analgesic efficacy of clodronate compared with placebo in patients with painful bone metastases from prostatic cancer. Anticancer Res, 17: 4717-4721, 1997.
71. Pelger RC, Hamdy NA, Zwinderman AH, Lycklama a Nijeholt AA, Papapoulos SE. Effect of the bisphosphonate olpadronate in patient with carcinoma of the prostate metastatic to the skeleton. Bone, 22: 403-408, 1998.
72. Heidenreich A, Hofmann R, Engelmann UH. The use of bisphosphonate for the palliative treatment of painful bone metastases due to hormone refractory prostate cancer. J Urol, 165: 136-140, 2001.
73. Heidenreich A, Elert A, Hofmann R. Ibandronate in the treatment of prostate cancer associated with painful osseous metastases. Prostate Cancer Prostatic Dis, 5: 231-235, 2002.
74. Ernst DS, Tannock IF, Venner PM, Winquist EW, Reyno L, Walker H, Ding K, Elliot C, Parulekar W. Randomized placebo controlled trial of mitoxantrone/prednisone and clodronate versus mitoxantrone/prednisone alone in patients with hormone refractory prostate cancer. (Abst) Proc Am Soc Cin Oncol 21: 705, 177a, 2002.

INDEX

D

E

F

G

H

I